ONE

S P L I T

Can you remember one

E

SPLIT- SECOND, that for better or worse, changed

C

your life? When you think of it, you could write

O

book; about the SPLIT-SECOND choices made,

N

or the happenstance for change.

D

BURNED ON MY MIND.

BY WINDY WYNN

ISBN 0-7414-3043-6

Published by:

INFINITY
PUBLISHING.COM

1094 New DeHaven Street, Suite 100
West Conshohocken, PA 19428-2713
Info@buybooksontheweb.com
www.buybooksontheweb.com
Toll-free (877) BUY BOOK
Local Phone (610) 941-9999
Fax (610) 941-9959

Printed in the United States of America

Printed on Recycled Paper

Published June 2006

SYNOPSIS

I was nearly electrocuted by touching a faulty elevator button. This book is for the thousands of brain injury patients, like myself, and their families. As I relive my struggle to overcome the physical problems and the prejudice shown; with dogged determination, I returned to some sort of normalcy. My story encourages others to find the ability to accept the things they can not change, and the strength to fight the ignorance, with the dignity to persevere. It will also enlighten the populace about the dangers of Electrical Current Burns, their treatment, and prevention.

BIOGRAPHY

This author has a real love of Nature and Human Nature. As a Registered Nurse, (working in such specialties as Neonatal ICU, CCU, and the ER) for the past thirty years, she has gained keen insight into Human Nature and our ability to survive tragedy, with the determination to fight our way back. Ah, the beauty of that human spirit!

SCUBA diving, photography, flying, and travel help her understand the solace of Nature. She likes to share her insight; through poetry, photography, and writing. Though, this will be a first-person-story of her brain injury and the struggle back.

FORWARD

THE AGONIZING AUTHOR.

Many a student will lay claim to this title, when pressed for the term paper. I dare say, none will know true agony, until their abilities (no matter how small they perceive them to be) are ripped away. You persevere, because so much is riding on it. This book is an important thesis on the gut-wrenching aftermath of the victims of post-traumatic neuropathy. I can only elaborate on the problems I encountered from my Near-Electrocution, due to a faulty elevator. As a nurse, I feel it my duty to educate the public; AND "The Profession," who seem to be left in the dark ages. When I touched that UP-button on the elevator, little did I know, I nearly went ***all the way up***. I'm lucky to be alive. That person; that personality which had taken years of learned coping mechanisms, was now, an empty shell. Your English term paper or my story might have taken two or three months, before this injury. You have handed in your term paper, been graded, and the task is finished. For me, those three months have turned into years. Let's explore the reasons:

Do you know how difficult it is to research material with **Short-term Memory Loss**? There is no hope for detail. Grab an important piece of information from the page and write it down, because you are not going to remember it, by the time you turn the page. When I am writing about actual events, I must depend on my Medical Logs… the notes the doctors asked me to write, so they could follow my progress. I would have to out-line the logs; make a list of the subject, and the date it happened.

With no memory, I needed a time-frame. I may have thought that I had covered the subject well, only to find there was more important information to come. At any rate, the *List of Subjects* got me started. Now, what chapter did I put that in? Or, had I covered that before? If I go back to read the chapters in search of a subject, I may forget the subject I was looking for. That symptom is what they call **Attention Deficit**. I can go in circles. Guidance in new coping mechanisms will help some; it was suggested that I put a table of contents on the front of each chapter. A little extreme? Not really. I numbered a 3x5 card and listed the subjects covered. I would then, attach them to the chapter. This helped somewhat, but some items were worth repeating in other context. With this *FOG*, every little hint would help; and the cards helped me identify and locate subjects I had already covered.

Let's add other aberrant nuisances. A student might glibly say that he can't think of a thing to write; how about, not being able to think, period? Or, how about loosing the ability to say or think of a word right in the middle of your sentence? You can't even think of a synonym! Not only was this a problem with my speech and thought, it was evident in my writing and typing. I would find sentences with words missing. **BUT THE BIGGY!** My right hand is slower than the left. You would not recognize the typed page. It looked like some sort of code. I can guarantee, there are no typed pages without mistakes, even to this day. What may have taken a normal person a few minutes, will have taken me twice the time. One point that cannot be emphasized enough, is the fact that I still have the same intelligence as before the accident; the pathways have been scarred and the messages and responses are slowed. If it seems we're walking in a daze, it's because we are! That does not make us idiots. (However, it has not said much for you, who do not understand.) The short-term memory has played heck with my retention of new material. Any new knowledge comes from hands-on experiences. (You can just imagine how many chapters have been lost to that big bad computer!) Everyday is like a new birth; I won't remember today, what happened yesterday. With the attention deficit, a simple story became a major project. This struggle is really ***unreal!*** It is a never-ending nightmare. My only hope came in acceptance. This was difficult for a "Perfectionist." The sentence structure and punctuation were never good enough. This entailed writing and rewriting untold times. I have finally accepted the fact that I can only do the best that my abilities will allow. My wish is for clarity. Perhaps, if you overlook my frailties, you can comprehend my candor. Our future lies in your understanding; then, ultimately, your tolerance. Believe me, we are hard enough on ourselves!

At first, friends and relatives would hear of my Near-Electrocution and think, "Wow, she's lucky to be alive!" (A year before, we had left them behind, in another state. They had not seen me on a day-to-day basis.) The next time they did see me, they expected me to be as sharp and witty as before. This was heartbreaking, because I expected the same thing EVERYDAY. But, it would not be. You could look at me and I appeared the same as I always was; there was no charred flesh, no obvious burn scars, nor was my hair singed-off. Therefore, one would assume, I was okay. With Electricity, the damage is often hidden inside. Your bodies electrical system (the nerve pathways) has been short-circuited. It took a while for friends to realize, **I WAS NOT ME!** Not the person I used to be. It would take time to regain my essence…that whole package which was me. As the years pass, there have been great improvements. Little by little, I will find myself; then, perhaps, **others will find me**. If not the old me, than the new improved model, who does the best they can, with what they have.

TABLE OF CONTENTS:

1. THE SPLIT SECOND 1
   "California Crazy" 11

2. A SHOCKING TURN-OF-EVENTS. 13
   "The Mystery Of The Living Dead" 23

3. THE SPIN CYCLE 25

4. IGNORANCE WAS OBVIOUS 37

5. SHOPPING, A WHOLE NEW WORLD. 53

6. FAULTY NERVE ENDINGS......................................73

7. ONLY A HEARTBEAT AWAY.................................89
   "So What ?!!!"..102

8. COPING MECHANISMS 111
   "Spin Cycle, Too" 132

9. SPIN CYCLE II 133
   "Mystery, Intrigue, Deceit and the Will to Survive". ..146

10. A REASON FOR STUBBORN PERSEVERANCE...147
    "Should I Clean It Up?!"..163

11. THOSE FIVE STAGES OF GRIEF. 165

12. RECYCLED..173

13. WHAT REALLY HAPPENED? 179
"Out of Body" 210

14. LIFE GOES ON. 213

15. I'VE COME A LONG WAY.......................................233
"Just For-The-Day" 251

16. MY RE-EVALUATION. 257

17. IN THE SCHEME OF THINGS..................................271
Life 280

18. POSTSCRIPT 283
Textures of My Life. 287
Now, I'm Retired!!!! 312

CHAPTER 1

THE SPLIT SECOND

THE SPLIT-SECOND.

I suppose every unusual happening occurs in a split-second. This is good. Otherwise, we would analyze it to death and mess up. We make wiser decisions when the adrenaline is rushing and we are standing-on-our-feet, facing-the-foe. All of life's experiences are but lessons to be learned for the future. We cannot do anything about the past, even that split-second, so you put it behind you and press forward. Most unusual things are exciting; yet, some excitement we feel we could do without:

I'm flying my plane through a restricted airspace. I had called the Base and received permission to do so. It was such a lovely day… just my plane and I, with all of nature's beauty for as far as the eyes could see. What a relaxing flight! In that split-second, four Phantom Jets turned on their wing-tips to avoid wiping out the whole lot, me included! Man! They were so close I could have spit in their eyes (had they not been moving so fast). The radio roared, "Who is flying in restricted airspace?" I shot back, "Who is flying in my airspace? I'm on an approved flight plan. You weren't even supposed to be flying maneuvers this afternoon!" Well, what was done, was done! Fortunately, life goes on… for all of us.

We're taking our private plane to Grand Cayman for a long weekend of S.C.U.B.A. A rather boring flight, once you get away from the land and the out-islands. Oh, you see an occasional tanker or cruise ship, but it's more like watching paint dry. (I'm taking this opportunity to break down my underwater camera and give it a good cleaning.) We can see clouds in the distance… probably Cuba. Did you ever notice how, even on a clear day, there will be clouds over a land mass? Interesting. We crossed the rocky coast of Cuba; on our approved flight plan to Cayman. It looked pretty much like any other island. There was nothing to see at this altitude, so I continued cleaning my camera; it lay on a towel in my lap, in a million pieces. As I looked up to rest my eyes, I saw a Cuban Mig out my window. As I turned my head to tell the pilot, I saw another Mig out his window. And there was another one above us. **"Unidentified aircraft approaching the Cuban coast. You are entering Cuban Airspace! Turn around and depart immediately!"** What are they talking about?? We crossed the Cuban coast ten minutes ago! The pilot had looked down at his radio and was busy changing to the Havana Tower frequency, when we noticed the Migs. My Buddy got on the radio to Havana Tower, identifying himself and reminding them that we were on an approved flight plan from Miami to Grand Cayman. He read the telegram giving us permission to over-fly Cuba, signed by the military attache. **NO RESPONSE TO OUR MESSAGE !!** Then, **"AIRCRFT ENTERING CUBAN AIRSPACE, DEPART IMMEDIATELY !! "** (Gee, was that our second warning?) I've always had this unwavering sense that justice shall prevail. Now, I'm a little uncomfortable. I'm remembering the rumors of private planes being forced down over Cuba, the occupants never heard of again. The planes were later found to be ferrying drugs from Columbia to Cuba, for distribution in the United States. Our pilot repeats his message; once again, reading the telegram from the attache. **AGAIN, NO RESPONSE !!** Then, like a guardian angel, "This is commercial flight so-and-so, at 25,000 feet. I understand you are having trouble raising Havana Tower. Stay on this frequency. I will relay your message and get back to you." That next couple of minutes of silent anticipation seemed hours. Then, strangely enough, Havana Tower came in loud and clear. They informed us that the attache who had given us permission to over-fly Cuba, was no longer in office. (There was a lot of purging going on at that time… and we're not talking bulimia here.) They were going to permit the over-flight, but we must maintain our flight path and take no pictures while over Cuban territory. We were to request over-flight previleges two days in advance of our return flight. (Oh, I am so sure we will be returning via Cuba!!! Isn't that like, "You put your left hand on the stove? That's a nasty burn. Now, put your right hand on the stove.") And "No problema," with the picture-taking. The camera is broken-down in my lap. I really hadn't seen anything worth the effort anyway. We were too high. The Migs had disappeared as quickly as they had appeared. Of course, THE MIGS! Now, that might have made an interesting picture! I remember the pilots were wearing those leather caps like the old Barnstormers used to wear. I'm told the *Goofy* headgear contained their microphones and receivers. Needless-to-say, we will be flying around Cuban Airspace on our return. So much for my Cuban experience! I can do without another MIGRAINE, for the rest of my life.

As an Air Ambulance Nurse, I had been detained in Central America for "trying to spirit a suspected terrorist bomber out of the country." **WHO, ME ?! I'm just a nurse, doing my job!** We were put-up in a hotel and asked to stay close until the matter was cleared-up. (So much for our Governments warning to keep *your passport on you, at all times*. **This Country would be holding our passports, for us!)** Our pilot contacted the boss, who in turn, kept our families informed. It would have been much easier on everyone, had we known more about our host-country, before the trip! Never a dull moment. Your imagination could just go wild. On the third day, the flight crew and passenger were given permission to leave. Finally! **Not so fast!** It took a while to convince the authorities that the Nurse was considered a part of the flight crew, on an Air Ambulance. At last, permission to leave. As our plane lifted off the runway, I knew that this was a pretty land with polite people. A land I would like to visit one day. I knew we were innocent and felt that my patient was innocent … there we go again … that faith that if you are in the right, justice will prevail! Boy, am I naïve! At altitude, you would never have known that there was fighting below; the days of the Contras and Sandinistas. From a distance, our world seemed at peace. The beauty was breathtaking. A simple experience like this, gives you a renewed appreciation for the good old U.S.A. It was good to be heading home. True, I had met El Presidente, who would go on to become a great leader of the whole Caribbean Basin. Such a gentleman! There were also Network Big-Shots and Reporters to remember. But, most of all, the ordinary people of a lovely land. Life is great!

Diving the cold, dark waters west of Mexico was a shock to one who had only dived warm waters. I had basked in the sun, while our slow boat carried us to the dive site. As my Buddy and I fell back into the dark waters, I became chilled. I indicated to my Buddy that I was cold and that this would be a short dive. He agreed and we started down. The waters were so dark, you couldn't see your hand in front of your face (at least, if you held your hand at arms length). Gee, It's amazing… the deeper we went, the warmer the water became; at a hundred feet, you could see forever. There were huge trees of Black Coral, swaying in the current, like great Weeping Willows. I felt the hand on my shoulder and looked my Buddy in the eyes. He smiled and signaled for us to go up. Yes, he was right. THE RAPTURE OF THE DEEP. I was narc'd out. Nitrogen Narcosis. I still had enough sense to realize what was happening, but it seemed so real! (Fortunately, ascending a few feet will clear your thoughts. That's why we dive with Buddies! Well, I've pulled his old butt out of the RAPTURE before. I could say "we're even" but actually, we were quite fortunate.) I was so affected, when we got back to the boat, I talked of diving the next day. "We could just drop down and snap off one of those Black Coral trees and come right back to the boat. It was only 125 feet deep. No problem. What great pictures we would have!" (Not to mention, we'd be rich!) I must have been badly Narc'd! Water does not get lighter the deeper one goes. It gets darker… and much,

much colder. I should not have dived in a chilled condition. If we are lucky, we live to learn from our experiences.

While visiting The Great Barrier Reef, we were going on a "shark-feed" dive. The crew went down and put bait along the reef. We divers all hunkered down close to the bottom to await the sharks. We were told that it would take a while for the sharks to sense the bait; be still and be patient. There will be nothing to see until the sharks come. My husband was busy trying out his new video camera. There was nothing to work with. He finally spotted a little snail on the bottom and was busy videotaping it, when the sharks appeared. The Divemaster signaled by waving his hand over his head. Obviously, he wanted us to go over to the next reef. I swam out into the open water and, as I reached the top of the reef, so did this big shark. Both of us stopped in mid-water, face to face. He looked down. Then, I looked down. Under my chin, lay half of a huge tuna. **Be my guest! It is all yours!** (After all of these years of diving, I can't believe I was trying to back-off by facing the shark, while using my flippers.... this, of course, would just propel you forward. At some point, I will have to turn and swim away. Maybe I can distract him, first.) I'm flashing my camera at him, in hopes of discouraging his advancement. I quickly decided that if he were going to bite me, I didn't want to see it coming. That uncomfortable feeling of the hair rising on the back of my neck, was with me. I turned and swam back to the others, who were still clinging close to the bottom, BUT getting great pictures. What depth perception I had given them... compare the size of this shark with the size of that brave *(idiot)* diver. Meanwhile, my husband was still videotaping the snail. I'm in a *Life and Death* situation here and he had missed the whole thing! I guess, I had hoped that he would have gotten my demise on tape, for shark research. I felt a chill and was ready to return to the boat. (All right! The waters of the world rose a bit that day.) Back on board, everyone wondered at my bravery and how I must have gotten some great pictures. Yeah, sure! I am so Cool! **ARE THEY KIDDING!!** I was fighting for survival! And the heck with pictures! Fisheyes are good, if we are speaking of camera lens. A piece of fish makes a nice meal, but not so great a picture. (Yes, I'm cool; probably a bit "Shocky.") Perhaps one of the other divers had gotten a picture of a whole shark. We didn't. (By the way, the darn snail was too small to even identify on video.) The Divemaster said that he had been signaling that the sharks were coming; **not** signaling for us to come. I had wondered why the rest of the group was so slow to follow their Divemaster. I just figured that they might have been a little intimidated by the appearance of sharks. Now, I know. I was the one with my signals crossed. Love them! The Aussies are great! Maybe we'll get our sign-language differences worked-out before we visit Australia again. That would help!

Our live-aboard arrived over the site of the wreck of the *YONGOLA* and we were given the usual orientation. You know, what to expect…the large fish, the sea snakes, etc. Did he say **sea snakes?!** One drop of their venom could kill everyone on board, but not to worry. They have to chew a hole in your skin to get the poison to you. Your wet suits will be thick enough to keep them away. They have little mouths. They are shy, but can be curious. If they bother you, just grab them by the tail and pull them off and swim away. (Boy! I don't know about anyone else, but this sure made me feel real comfortable. Since I only wear Lycra Skins, that shouldn't take more than a tiny nibble, even with their little mouths.) The only time you might see one, is when he is coming to the surface for air. Well, that was certainly an interesting orientation. We probably won't even see one. A picture would be nice, though. My husband (the straightman) is the videographer, while I take stills. Like most divers, we enter the water with our hands full of cameras and strobes. I keep my camera in the *off-position* until I reach the dive site; it takes a while for the flash to cycle. As we worked our way down the anchor line, I looked up to see this large Sea Snake weaving its way to the surface… around my husband's leg, around his waist, around his chest, around his neck, and then to the surface. All the time, I am screeching and pointing; trying to tell him to take video. He is looking everywhere, but at the snake. It seems his wet suit had protected him from all sensation. I don't know how to explain his "far-sightedness." When we returned to the boat and I told him about the snake, he couldn't believe it. He hadn't seen a thing. (Come to think of it, it was probably one of those *Blessings in Disguise.* Videography can be demanding. A snake may have been too much, after practicing on a snail.) I was too *thin-skinned* to mess with the snake, myself. The only other snake I saw, was down below, going into a hole. They say a picture is worth a thousand words. Alas! A picture of a flat tail, like a piece of a shark, says nothing.

One morning, I made a dive with a dive-buddy from New Zealand. We did the usual pre-dive talk about our dive plan and signals. Everything was going as planned, until he signaled we should return to the boat. I had noticed his checking my air supply gauge more frequently than usual; but, his supply was fine, and my supply was fine. What was his problem?! Before ascending, we agreed on a three-minute *hang-time*. Now, he is signaling "Three, at three." (What does he mean…three at three?) This is no time to quibble. He can just go up to three feet, if he wants to. We don't really need a "stop" to be safe. We hadn't even come close to the Tables. After all, I had been preaching about the benefits of hang-time, for years. I learned it from being so good on air, that I would hang back in the water and let everyone else onboard ahead of me. The other divers would be "bushed" for the next dive, while I would feel fresh-as-a-daisy and raring-to-go. Even to this day, I won't push my times or depths. And, I still advocate hang-times for every dive; you just feel more refreshed. I went to my ten-foot depth and, strangely enough, I was hanging face-to-face with my Buddy. He had come to his senses. As I came out of the water, he frantically helped me out of my tank and was amazed that I had <u>any</u> air left. What was his problem?! As a woman, I could usually do a two-tank-dive on a single 50 tank of air. I suppose we might have saved him some gray hair and saved both of us a longer dive on the great Yongola Wreck, had we just remembered the apothecary/metric equivalencies. So, ten feet would be about three meters. My Buddy suddenly appeared brilliant, next to me. Proving, sometimes you need to learn the language, even in an English-speaking country. Now, if any of you blokes have pictures of this hapless diver with sharks, how about sending me one?

Many things happen in a flash: You laugh at the fish that got away, (or the sea snake.) Wonder over the *Goofy* caps or at being an unwilling participant in some Air Force maneuver. Appreciate the help of the ordinary people in a foreign land. All the while, you know how incredibly lucky you are. You drink in the experience and become a better person. I enjoy my life and have always said that **"Life is for Living!"** You should live each day to the fullest. One never knows what tomorrow brings.... you could be hit by a MACK Truck. If I die young, (some of you will say, "too late.") don't cry for me. I will have *lived* more than a person of a hundred and three. So, we go on seeking new and exciting adventures to fill our spirits with joy. There are so many wonders of this world and so many fabulous people yet to meet. I love nature and I love human nature.

When it became evident we would be moving cross-country to follow his job, my husband and I looked at it all as "*just another great adventure*." What a beautiful place! We can hardly wait to get started. This will not be a simple vacation to share with friends and family. This is a life-changing experience; vacations become a chance to visit friends and family. We look forward to showing them the wonders of this great state. Come on out!

Our first Spring was like stepping into a Monet. (Perhaps, A Woman With a Parasol visiting the Garden at Giverny.) The yards were laced with so many beautiful flowers; and, the blooming trees were spilling forth their glory everywhere. Suddenly, and so completely, the Ice Plants covered the banks of the freeways, as if Mother Nature had waved her magic wand. They were breathtaking. Scores of wild flowers stole your attention away from the teaming traffic, giving you peace. The sun danced across the fields of bright yellow mustard. The hills had turned deep emerald green from the winter rains, which enhanced the bold white windmills spinning in the clear blue sky. The flyways were filled with birds of all colors; like one giant commercial, *their songs presenting us SPRING.* I must admit; I bought into this commercial. I couldn't help it. As the Robin Red Breast must sing his song, or his breast would surely burst, I had to express my joy, also. Here is the ditty I would call:

CALIFORNIA CRAZY

The daffodils are *daffy*.
The woods are *going wild.*
The hills are *green with envy* of
the mustard-colored fields.
The trees are *blooming idiots*, but
what has wrought these things?
Has the whole darn world *gone mad*, or
is it simply SPRING?

Forgive me. It must have been the Spring Fever. This place is truly that *Piece of Heaven on Earth*!

Sure, my friends tease me about my thoughts on HISTORY. In high school, my History Teacher had asked why I was not enthusiastic about the subject.... "Those who do not study the past, are destined to repeat their mistakes." Like every Senior, **I didn't want to read about history.... I WANTED TO MAKE HISTORY!** Every time something out of the ordinary happens to me, my friends claim that it is *payback* time. I should have given history its rightful place. Instead of cramming for a test; now, I'm scrambling to regroup after each challenge. Oh well, making your own personal history can be beautiful...... most of the time. Sometimes, those things which happen in a split-second, will be the things you find most challenging. The unexpected happenings, which were not planned for, may take added effort and time. But, this is life. And we grow from "Life."

CHAPTER 2

A SHOCKING TURN-OF-EVENTS.

A SHOCKING TURN-OF-EVENTS...

I remember thinking that I was going to get-off on time tonight. This is great! We seldom get out the door on time, working a busy Emergency Room. If the Incoming Phone doesn't ring within the next fifteen minutes, we're out of here! I was already having visions of all sorts of extra time to "roll around" tonight. I will probably be home before my husband, if we get out on time. I was deep in thought, as we rushed the patient to CCU for observation. As we approached the elevator, the EMT stopped pushing and took her hand off of the back of the gurney. I pulled up to the elevator, with one hand between the rails of the gurney, resting on the Life-Pac; I reached to touch the "UP" button. **C R A C K !!** My body stiffened, my neck arched back, and my hands flew straight up, like someone being defibrillated without a backboard. There was a quick flash in my eyes, then everything went black; like being in a dark cave with a flashlight, when the flashlight goes out. My eyes were open, but everything was pitch black. There was intense heat in both arms, across my chest, and the back of my brain. There was warmth on my inner thighs. I feel myself falling.... It is like my feet are glued flat against the floor; yet, I'm falling from the ankles up. My ankles are like jelly! I've heard of being weak-kneed, but never weak-ankled.

Though I couldn't see, I was reaching for anything, to break my fall. I was able to catch myself, on the way down; one hand on the mattress of the gurney and one hand on the floor. As I pulled myself up, I realized that the warmth between my legs had been an incontinence of urine... I'm soaked! (Just like a nurse ...never time to empty the bladder! There must have been a gallon!) I smell singed hair, but I don't see any. Fortunately, <u>I can see</u> again. Thank God! My ears feel burnt. The EMT tells me that they are bright red, but the skin is intact. I just feel.... in a stupor. Everything is in slow-motion; I'm hearing, but not comprehending as quickly; I'm seeing, but recognition is slowed. Nothing is making sense! My hands are numb, but I can still make use of them.

The poor EMT is in a tight place...she could hardly leave a cardiac patient in the hall and take me back to the ER. She couldn't leave me unattended. After assessing my abilities, she made the decision to take the patient on to the Unit, with me following, like a little puppy. I was of no help. (Fortunately, the patient was a tiny little man and not an inch of him was touching the gurney at the time. There may have been an entirely different outcome, had he been.) We returned to the ER, where the EMT reported what had happened, got me a clean pair of scrubs, and helped me with the accident report. I was a useless mess. I knew what had happened, but couldn't put it into words. I guess someone could see I needed assistance, when I wrote that I had received a shot from the elevator.

* * * * * * *

THE AFTERMATH:

WEAK AND DAZED! How can I explain what I'm feeling? The back of my brain feels like it is being bathed in hot water, and it's as if someone was pressing their hands against the back of my head. Such pressure!

BURNING UNDER THE RIBCAGE feels like a thick piece of plastic lining that has been infused with laser heat. NO PAIN…in fact, NO FEELING AT ALL under the ribs. I surmise the lungs are functioning well. I am still breathing; which means the chest rises and falls. I can see it, though I can't feel it. I feel no air entering the nostrils or flowing into the lungs. It seems there is an obstruction in the right side of the nose. If I close-off the right nostril and take a breath, the chest rises. If I close-off the left nostril and take a breath, the chest does not rise. (Later, when I blew my nose, there was a huge blood clot. Ah, the secret of that smell of singed hair. It must have been the hair in my nose.)

Everything remains in "SLOW MOTION." I can hear, but it takes a while for my brain to decipher the information and react. I find that I am at-a-loss-for-words. Perhaps if I'm quiet, no one will notice.

The RED EARS feel like a severe sunburn at the tops; no itching or red face, just bright red ears. They burn like fire!

I feel my pulse and my heart is racing. I am just so drained! So weak!

EVERYTHING HAD HAPPENED SO FAST….that so-called **SPLIT-SECOND** really does exist! More like a nano-second.

* * * * * * *

WHAT'S HAPPENING, HERE? As far as I can see, NOTHING! I'm left alone, to fend for myself. If my heart stopped, would they even notice? (So much for the safety of the Emergency Room!) If I think I'm having trouble comprehending what is going on, think of the staff. (AND, as far as I know, none of them have had a brain injury!) They really haven't a clue! No one understood the possible effects of an Electrical Current Burn.

Everything is in "Slow Motion." There was no time for the ER doctor to examine me. I was just a nurse... an employee. Nothing more. Besides, there were *more pressing matters*: two patients complaining of chest pain were brought in, shortly after the change of shifts. All attention was on them. The on-coming charge nurse insisted that I help, even if I had had an injury and had already clocked out... "I would be paid over-time." She hadn't a clue! Like the little puppy following commands, I forced myself out of the chair and into the Cardiac Room to help. Fortunately, the other nurse sensed my problem and instructed me to return to the nursing station. **My condition was so obvious!** I looked like a deer caught in the headlights, for crying out loud! Every time the ER doctor rushed by, he would ask how I felt. (What do I know? It takes me 20 minutes to decipher the information and come up with an answer.) The ER was busy and I was extremely weak and tired. I would seek the doctor and ask if he was going to get an EKG on me. "Sure, if you want one," he replied. They played around with my EKG's, for what seemed an hour, adjusting the amplitude, until they were able to get a reading that didn't look like a *straight-line.* I kept telling them that I was alive; "I'm talking to you." The Doc listened to my symptoms, but really hadn't heard me. AFTER ALL, THERE APPEARED TO BE NO OBVIOUS INJURY!! So, three hours after the mishap, I drove myself home that early morning, even though I could not think clearly. I was incapable of making that decision on my own, and should never have been behind the wheel of a car. I've had a **TRAUMATIC BRAIN INJURY!** (As time goes by, I would find *many* who *would listen, but not really hear.* This would become so EXTREMELY FRUSTRATING !! Yet, what can I do? <u>They will not hear</u>.)

There are few cars on the freeway at 2:30 AM. That is fortunate, 'cause I feel like a Zombie. I feel like a hollow shell. Though I am part American Indian, I feel like an American Indian Drum; skin pulled tightly over a void of bones. My brain has been fried and my insides are missing (or so it seems… I can't feel them!) I wonder if Zombies drive cars. If there was an impending accident, how long would it take for me to react? I don't know. I just kept driving, hoping to be home before anything could happen. If there was an accident, who would be aware of my condition? I've had patients in the ER before, who had had electrical shocks; I realized that most of the injury was on the inside. I wonder why the ER Staff had not recognized that fact, in my case.

Eventually, I understood, most really hadn't a clue. If you are raised in a family of auto mechanics, you would know more than the average person, about cars. As the daughter of an electrician, I was better informed than most, regarding the workings of electricity. Then again, perhaps they had not seen as many shock patients as I. I've been in this business for more years than I would care to admit. I had to beg for the EKG; yet, I wonder why they had not gotten blood and urine tests, also. Baselines to cover their bases. My treatment, or lack thereof, seemed negligent. Still, it is difficult to catch a problem you cannot see; and there were no huge hunks of charred flesh hanging from my bones, my hair was not singed off, and it was way past my bedtime so why wouldn't I be like a Zombie?! It occurred to me that **NOBODY KNOWS!!**

When I got home, my husband was furious that the hospital had sent me home in such a condition…I, on the other hand, just wanted to get some sleep. He wanted to take me back to the hospital and let them explain how they could send a patient home, in that condition. I refused, stating that by morning, I would be fine. (I've always been that *Cockeyed Optimist* you read about.) By the time I climbed the stairs, my pulse was 140. I will have to rest before I take my shower. I'm glad I had bathed when I changed my scrubs, because I went into such a deep sleep my husband couldn't awaken me. He just watched me through the night; checking my respirations and pulse, both shallow.

Well, no overnight miracles! I'm pretty much the same. This morning, my back feels like it has a bad sunburn, but we see no burned skin; another obvious internal injury. It probably has something to do with that *burned plastic lining* under my ribs. At the same time, I have pressure over my kidneys, much like the pressure on the back of my head. Maybe, if I just get moving, my head will clear and these other symptoms will disappear.

The drive to work was very exhausting and I called the Nursing Supervisor to let her know that I would not be able to work, in this condition. I told her that I was still weak from the SHOCK; I have tachycardia, can't think clearly, everything is in slow-motion, and it's difficult for me to just follow what is being said or what was going on. She said that I would have to stay for four hours, regardless; until she could find someone else to come in. Once again, *someone was listening, but not really hearing.* I triaged colds and broken bones until the replacement came on duty. That is pretty safe, even for a challenged nurse. Why can't I think clearly? It's been nearly a day! My ears keep turning red, it feels like someone has their hands on the back of my head, there is pain on the top of the right side of my head, and the cheeks around my eyes are numb. No wonder I can't think clearly. It's like a constant nag. I'm just sitting here at the Triage Desk, but

I'm so tired. Every time I make a sudden move, my pulse shoots up over a hundred. I get short-of-breath, just walking across the room. (Thank goodness, it is a slow night, so far.)

Boy! This is not normal for me; I was born running, and never stopped. **I don't understand.** I'm in great shape. I have always done the mat exercises daily, to assure good strong muscle tone and condition; something a nurse needs to prevent back injuries. I ride my stationary bike five miles every morning. Then, I ride my mountain bike another five miles before going to work, where I can run for another eight or ten hours. **Why can't I shake this?!** I seem to be getting worse, not better. Maybe, the drive to work, was just too much, too soon. I'll rest tomorrow. I just have a Nursing Up-Date Class in the morning. Surely, I'll be back to normal, by then. I do notice spatter burns on both hands today. The pattern is the same on both sides: from the webs of my thumbs and index fingers, up the arms three inches past the wrists. And, of course, the hair was singed off of these areas.

I almost feel guilty about complaining. It could have been much worse. **I might have died!** With all the heat across the back of my head, I am thankful that I can still see. And though I am numb under my ribcage, I am still breathing. I take pleasure in watching my chest rise and fall. (Something you could normally feel, but not now.) The *Cockeyed Optimist* is beginning to sound like everyone else. If I can see, if I can breathe, if I can function (never mind, to what degree)...then I must be alright! No! No! No! Why can't I think? **I feel like an entity from another world.** Surely, a Zombie! I must be **the living dead!** I feel as though my very soul is missing. **I am not ME!** I have a strong Faith in God and I know He loves me and will take care of me. It's a good thing, because I can't concentrate long enough to pray. What can I use for coping? I feel a need to connect with others, in order to make a connection with ***This World***. You would be surprised how different things seem, when you can not feel your lungs, your heart, or your insides. Yes, there is a definite connection between those so-called *"feelings"* and your heart. That warm glow is gone. Inside, I'm cold; it seems as if my very core is missing. **I AM SO EMPTY !** (Maybe tomorrow!)

By the third day, I am beginning to think that this is all going to take a little longer than I had anticipated. I don't know why I attended this Nursing Up-Date Class. I am not absorbing any of this information! When will the fog clear? This may take a few more days. My whole life is surreal! Everything is still in "Slow Motion." Just everything stopped with the push of a button. A simple split-second has completely rearranged my very being. I don't like this feeling. I must try to concentrate! I know I need to clear my head, but things seem to be getting worse. How can this be happening? Perhaps, when the burning pressure eases from the back of my head… Then, there is that "sunburn" feeling across my back. The red ears and numb hands are a part of the problem, also. I understand that burns feel worse before they feel better; but, it feels like a couple of red hot coals are burning deep in my skull. It could take a week or two, before my head clears and this "Slow Motion" goes away. Perhaps, a little longer.

After two weeks, the burning spots in the skull have turned into white hot embers; waiting to spring forth on the slightest whim. **I am walking a tightrope, here!** Unsure of my destiny. (Yes, I'll admit, I've always been impatient. I can't be bothered with this inconvenience. Let's get over it, already! Then guilt kicks in, and I remind myself how lucky I am to have survived. **I will learn patience**!) As the days turned into weeks, weeks into months, and months into years; I never gave up hope, but I had questions …when will I ever?…why can't I?…what can I do?… How can I help? …How long will it be?…How much longer will it be? Will I ever?… Can I expect more improvement? I will learn many things from this experience. Teach me to live with my disabilities. Make me strong enough to endure. Help me to help others. Recycle my abilities to cover my disabilities. **Make me happy with the "Me," that will be**.

THE MYSTERY OF THE LIVING DEAD.

WHERE IS MY SOUL? HAS IT GONE TO REST?

EVERYTHING SEEMS EMPTY, WITHIN MY BREAST.

I HAVE BECOME CAPTIVE IN THIS FOREIGN LAND.

LISTENING TO CALLS, I DON'T UNDERSTAND.

I'M WALKING THROUGH SWAMPS OF SPANISH MOSS,

THE FOG IS SO THICK, I FEAR THAT I'M LOST.

THE QUICKSAND SURROUNDS ME. I'M WALKING WITH CARE.

YET, KNOWING I'M HELPLESS; I'VE BEEN STRIPPED BARE.

MY WORLD IS FULL OF DANGER, FROM EVERY DIMENSION.

THE VIPERS STAND READY, RELEASING THEIR VENOM.

I'M FIGHTING ALLIGATORS, I CAN NOT SEE.

WONDERING, WHAT WILL BECOME OF ME?

HOW COULD THIS HAPPEN? I DON'T UNDERSTAND.

EACH DAY, MY HORROR STARTS OVER AGAIN.

CHAPTER 3

THE SPIN CYCLE

THE SPIN CYCLE...

The Company was working overtime, to put a spin on this SHOCK.!!!! The pecking system dictates that the underlings "smooth-over" anything that might make the Hospital look bad or cost money. They pulled out all stops! (Not to fix the problem, but to C.Y.A.)

Though many had received ***shocks*** from that elevator before my Near-Electrocution, and many would receive ***shocks*** after; the word was out that a nurse had received a *static electric shock* while transporting a patient to the floor. Therefore, they suggested that you "wear clothing of all natural fibers, rubber gloves, and shoe covers before transporting patients to the floor. Pushing the gurney over carpeting and touching the elevator button could cause static electricity." Does this sound logical? When was the last time you were cautioned about your apparel, before touching an elevator button, in a public building; or any building? Then, there was still this one little fact: <u>there is no carpeting</u> on the floor between the ER and the elevators! **IS ANYONE BUYING THIS?! I DON'T THINK SO!** Well, that could be a problem; so, there was a word-of-mouth campaign... "She lived in Florida for years and really doesn't understand what static electricity is all about." Even if Florida were some magic land, which never possessed conditions conducive to static electricity, **the peons know** that there are million of air-conditioned homes with nylon wall-to-wall carpeting. (Actually, I grew up in the Midwest, and it seems I received more static electric zaps in Florida than I ever did as a child.) Our only "*Magic*" in Florida is at Disney World!

I especially liked the campaign of how "the poor dear was so frightened, she wet her pants." Boy, did they ever waste that wildcard on the wrong person! I have no fear! Believe me, my life has been a little more eventful than to whine about a little *static electricity.* I've had some unusual experiences, but I've never.... well, the waters of the world did rise one time... but you couldn't say I wet my pants. They were already wet, and I was cold. Anyway, it is still my theory about not being able to change the past, which negates the wet pants story. As if the traumas weren't bad enough: I'm like a Zombie, I have delayed responses, everything is in slow motion and I have difficulty just understanding what is going on. This FOG *of grogginess* is over-powering. Other shock-related injuries haven't helped much, either: My head burns and the pressure is so great, I feel it will pop; I'm getting very little sleep, thanks to the "sunburn" across my back; and the tachycardia makes me weak. Now, on top of that, I must put up with all of this **SPIN.** My inhibitions are down. My coping is like that of a child. The pity had gotten so thick, I called my Union Representative, to arrange a meeting with management, in order to clear-the-air and set the record straight. I wanted to discuss this reality, the facts released, and the fallacies and degradation to stop. These people should not be teasing me, but trying to help. I'm being set-up and I should not be called upon to answer idiotic questions of doubt that anything ever happened. (Those who questioned most, became believers; when they too, would receive Shocks.)

Over the years, it has never ceased to amaze me: how, a Company will insist on an IQ Test, as a condition of employment; then, once hired, they expect everyone to become apathetic idiots, incapable of an original thought. It's as if we lived in the Middle Ages, where the Emperor tells the peasants what to believe. Talk about "**Illusions of grandeur**"!!! Or, should we say, Illusions of grander.... "I'm grander than you. I'm a smart boss, and you are dumb peons. If it weren't for me, this empire would crumble. I'm very important, so I will take a 30% raise and give a **great** party to let everyone know how **great** I am." Three months later, the peons get the talk about how "the company will have to tighten-its-belt. Sure, it will mean a cutback. Some will loose their jobs, but the company can survive." **DO YOU THINK THE PEONS ARE BUYING THIS?** On a Midwestern farm, you might hear, "What a crock-of-crap!" My favorite was "Bull Hockey." Somehow, when we shortened it to "Bull!" or "What a Crock!" it seemed nicer. A civil person would simply say, "I am not buying that!" The sophisticated person would merely say, "Amazing." Should we bother telling them; how we, the common people, are quite capable of logical thinking and using common sense? Why bother? They are so full of themselves they would never believe it. Logic and common sense seems to escape them. (Besides, who wants to tell the Emperor he's naked?) Did someone say, *Peters' Principle?* Have you noticed, the higher some climb the ladder, the looser their rungs?

For others of the same ilk: We laugh at them, yet they annoy us when they cut into other programs. I'm speaking of the News Anchors who actually believe that John Q. Public cares, one iota, about their personal opinions on the problems of the world. Here's a real FLASH for you! **We don't care**! A taxi driver delivers you to your destination. That's his job. That's what he gets paid for. A ditch digger can take his machine and dig a hole to precise measurements. That's his job. That's what he gets paid to do. A cleaning woman can work wonders on a dirty house. That's her job. That's what she gets paid to do. A pilot flies a plane. That's his job. That is what he gets paid to do. All are experts at their own particular job. (Many CEO's couldn't find their way out of a board room, much less drive a taxi to its' destination. Thank God, they don't fly the airplane!) A News Anchor is hired to deliver the news...*parrot the words*. Try doing the job you are paid to do. Please, don't waste our time with your latest "take on the news." Just the facts, **please!!!!!** (Such arrogance!) I'm sure you're convinced that your viewers are such idiots, they really can't comprehend what you are trying to say, so you repeat the same paragraph over and over again; days, weeks, and months on end. If this is the case, **maybe you're in the wrong business!** We *"Idiots"* really are interested in what goes on in the rest of the world. The Pope visited Cuba, but who would know? Give us the News; you know, something that is NEW! Keep your personal political agenda to yourselves, and leave us time for some Ball Games and Soaps. Don't advertise World News, if you are not going to "mouth" world news. (At least, we've all learned a lot about *"Smoke and Mirrors."*) We should all do our individual jobs to the best of our ability. And, a writer should stick to writing! And so, back to my reality**. The Meeting!**

Now, **the Company is trying to blame everyone and everything else.** 1. Perhaps a bolt of **lightening** entered the elevator shaft. Though there were no storms in the area that night, lightening could travel thirty miles. 2. They had their maintenance representative explain that the Hospital had checked the **elevators** and had found no shorts or other problems. (Strange. I had heard stories about personnel receiving shocks in the O.R., also. It was right across the hall from the elevators. I guess they were just stories. Though, some would recall that the elevator certificate was a month over-due inspection, when this thing happened to me. Would it have made a difference? We doubt it.) I was told that I could not sue the elevator company, because the hospital had changed to their own maintenance department for up-keep and inspections. And, of course, in this *no-fault state,* you cannot sue your employer, if you are hurt on the job. (Even if it was caused by an on-going problem of continued negligence.) 3. Perhaps I had received a shock from a faulty **cardiac monitor**, which I had been touching. A representative of the company that had manufactured the monitor, insisted that it could not have fired without someone pushing the button, and that they had found no defects. (Gee, do you think that the shock from the faulty elevator could have caused the monitor to fire? No, Wait!

The lightening came down the elevator shaft, causing a faulty elevator button, which fired the monitor! Yeah, that's the ticket! A three-way shock! That way, no one is to blame. About as believable as any of the other theories.) So, we are left with the old *lightening down the elevator shaft again*. How many times do you think lightening will collect in the same elevator shaft?! It must have been many, 'cause so many people had received those *static electric shocks.* **(Does this sound like I'M GETTING-THE-SHAFT?!)** The handwriting was on the wall. Even in my fragile state, it seemed clear to me, that the Company would do anything to avoid taking responsibility for their negligence. We sensed an air of arrogance here, also.

Struggling on, the Company made my life as miserable as they possibly could. As I look back, I wonder if they changed insurance carriers, because their present carrier wanted to settle. Maybe, their present carrier simply changed their name, to get out-from-under the possibility of a major pay-out. It happens. Or, the carrier may have found them to be too great a risk; these faulty elevators, could kill someone. I don't pretend to know the answer to that, but I do know that I was sent on wild goose chases all over creation, examined by many of their doctors, lied to by their representatives, and denied rightful compensation. My husband and I had thought it strange, I should receive piddling sums for small incidents. (Might it make them appear honorable?) We certainly hadn't expected them to give me a penny for little injuries, since they had ignored my Near-Electrocution! Tennis elbows were minor, compared to these Electrical Current Burns. We understood fully, why they had not given me, so much as a dollar in settlement. That would mean that they were accepting responsibility for the injury, and would have had to provide the compensation, I should be receiving each month. There was no way this would happen! **There is no honor among thieves**.

In the meantime, just two and a half months after the Near-Electrocution, I received a letter informing me that they would pay me for the days I had missed work and all medical bills, up to that date; but they felt that there would be no further medical treatment necessary and that they would not authorize any further medical care.... even though, they had not yet received all of the reports from the many doctors. (My husband and I have been paying the on-going medical bills since.) I liked the form letters I received, reminding me I could call, if I had questions. Well, I think I have a lot of questions, but I haven't the ability to ask them or to retain the information I would be given. A Workers Comp form letter assured me that I had the right to hire a lawyer. Sure! Hiring a lawyer would be hard enough a task; couldn't you just see that case? I don't remember or retain information, so the poor guy would have to rely on my medical log. I can tell you, it is long and it is boring. Don't waste our time. Lawyers don't see any money in my case; "You cannot sue your employer for injuries, in this State." The one lawyer I hired, for reimbursement of the mileage incurred, was a farce. Like most people, he couldn't be bothered with details of other issues; just get the mileage and close the case. He knew that I would not be able to assist; I wouldn't know the difference anyway, because I won't remember anything. Ignorance abounds! He couldn't understand my type of "*amnesia*." After all, I did remember a few things, so I must be okay. Forget about asking for compensation. I suppose these people feel like, if you walk away alive, you don't warrant compensation benefits for the disabilities and the medical bills that remain. I feel it is still a male/female situation. You know, if this were a man, more effort would have gone into doing the right thing. Paranoia? Perhaps, but my whole case was taken as lightly as a broken fingernail. Yet, here I am, a broken life. He'll get his money. Besides, this guy was busy playing with his toys: He had a picture on the wall. The first time I was there, nothing was said. My notes reminded me of the next time I was there; he had me racking-my-brain, as he showed me how to see the *Hidden Indians* in the field. "Hold your head still and don't blink your eyes, and you'll see them." It took so long for me to see the illusion, that it was tiring. These games just make my head pain and pressure worse. (Does this guy get paid by the hour?) When I was there for a deposition, he started playing the same little game. He asked me to tell the other man that I'd seen the Indians… "Look closely, they are there," I replied. The two men left the room for a minute. I told the transcriber: "I don't see any Indians in that picture today. I don't remember what they looked like, anyway; but I had seen them once. To tell the truth, I think he has a "like" picture in the closet, and he switches them. Or, it could be painted with glass beads; which will only show up, when the light is on." We laughed, and they were back. He definitely gets paid by the hour! I always felt that my visits to his office were a waste of time. It's easy to see, **the disabled are** not represented, but rather, **taken advantage of.** At least, he was willing to be an official-looking name on the request for reimbursement. Most lawyers refused; saying they couldn't take a case like this. Too time-consuming, with no hope of a successful out-come.

Every W/C doctor I had to see became an ordeal. The Company would submit a list of three names for us to choose from. Then, THEY made the appointments and notified us. (That didn't mean that the doctors' office knew about the appointment… "Everything takes time." And my husband and I pondered the fact that the only pre-requisite for a W/C doctor to qualify, was the fact that the distance traveled must be, at least, 150-200 miles. Even then, you might arrive for an appointment, only to find that no one had ever heard of you.) We were convinced that their effort to control our lives was their method of making the problem "go away." The pummeling had finally worn us down. My husband is just one person; these added responsibilities are just too much for him to continue. Besides, what could one expect, in this situation? W/C Insurance Company, W/C Doctors, with W/C Lawyers, in a W/C Court, with a W/C Judge. **Can**

we all say KANGAROO?! We were so sick-to-death over our treatment, that we would sign anything to get them to leave us alone. (And, wasn't that their ploy, all along?!) It was all he could do, to simply follow my condition. I'm **in this FOG**, so my husband is my sole guardian and advocate. I told the lawyer that we would sign, but they should be sure to let Workers Comp know that we could not lie, and that we did not agree with their findings. The attorney told us that we would have to sign the settlement, as is, if we wanted them to leave us alone. Though we all knew that there were permanent disabilities, I doubt that our protest was ever heard. We are just numbers.

Three years after the fact, I was presented with a **settlement check** for my *tennis elbows*; which were injured while lifting a patient to a stretcher, when his heavy leg caught the edge of the mattress, stopping the momentum. Sure, the tennis elbows will always bother me, on occasion; but the **Near-Electrocution** will be forever!!! **Nothing would be allowed for these Disabilities!!** We especially liked the slick way they slipped the no settlement for the SHOCK in between minor issues; they should be in politics. (I am finding all sorts of surprises in my files, since the *FOG* lifted. Of course, I don't remember seeing these things before. But then, that's one of the problems, isn't it? I don't remember! As I look them over, I knew I would not have understood them, at the time; though, I fully understand this rip-off, six years later.)

My poor husband! He had to take care of me, direct my well-being, encourage me, interpret letters, see to my doctor appointments and medication, PLUS hold down a full-time job. With our Family and Friends in a distant State, he had no help. What a saint! He really is strong and he really is SOMETHING SPECIAL. He does not deserve to suffer this harassment. On top of our lives being turned upside-down, we had to fight for payment of the medical bills and fight for reimbursement of mileage from the Company. Even silly little things like that! Our insurance didn't want to pay, because they knew that the medical problems were job-related. The Hospital was evading their responsibilities. The Company had become a **S**elect **C**ommittee **R**estricting **E**mployee **W**ages, while **U**ndermining their character. I'm sure you know what we called them, for short. The Gang!

While visiting the Employee Health Doctor for a respiratory problem, I was surprised to learn that he had never heard of my SHOCK and could not find anything relating to it, in my file. This is four years after the fact. AMAZING! You would think that even a *static electric shock* would wind up in my file, after my having been seen by an army of doctors. (It wasn't until a male nurse temporarily lost the use of his right arm, that they finally replaced the elevators. **What does that say?!!)**

As we're reminded, time and again, this is a "No-Fault State." Meaning, you cannot sue your employer, if you are hurt on the job. **The real problem with this is it leaves others in danger of injury.** I wanted OSHA brought in, but was given such a GUILT TRIP: "Sure, you could bring in OSHA, but do you really want to be responsible for all of your friends losing their jobs and the community losing a hospital that has served this community for 35 years?" In this *FOG of confusion*, I can't think straight. I certainly couldn't fight for any cause, in my condition. It was obvious there would be no OSHA! (Before this Near-Electrocution, you could have bet on my calling in OSHA, to protect my friends and the community. Not now. I am in such a fog… nothing makes much sense.) Every time I see a program on fraudulent insurance claims, I wonder when they are going to do a piece on the fraudulent Company Scams. We won't hold our breath. If a person can be taken advantage of, they will be. I could not help myself. They were quite aware of this fact. I am at their mercy, and **I FEEL SO HELPLESS!** I'm sure there are others who could not think clearly (due to concussions, traumatic neuropathy of strokes, or whatever), who are being denied their right to disability benefits. No-Fault leads to more Workers Comp abuse and continued negligence. What incentive do they have, to fix the problem?

With my childish feelings, I would find myself wishing that others could experience my symptoms—just for a short while—so they could understand all I was going through. Sounds like an eight-year-old, doesn't it?! Perhaps, this book will give you an idea of what we face daily. People are kinder, when they can see your disability; while, they don't understand or tolerate something they cannot see.

** (COULD YOU FIND THE **ATTENTION DEFICIT**?) When I read through these first few chapters, I was tempted to revise them; but, I am trying to write about "*what a person feels, during these times*." Bear with me. It is a constant struggle to keep focused on one subject, while writing this book. I will do the best that my abilities will allow; meanwhile, enjoy the variety. Take a break from the heartbreak. Reflect on the lighter side.

CHAPTER 4

IGNORANCE

WAS OBVIOUS

IGNORANCE WAS OBVIOUS.

Even in shock, I understood the ER doctor should have been getting an EKG and a urine test, at the least. He was busy with a couple of "chest pain" patients and really didn't concern himself with someone who looked okay. I was in shock. I was wiped-out. I just wanted to crawl into my bed and go to sleep. (In the hopes, that in the morning, this will have been just a bad dream.) After waiting at the nursing station for 2 or 3 hours, I finally had *gall enough* to ask the doctor if he was going to do any test. If not, "I want to go home." He said, if I wanted one, he would get an EKG. It was done, after the fact. **First aid dictates** that all cases of electrical trauma should be **treated in the Hospital**, to watch Cardiac Rhythm, get urinalysis and blood tests to check for internal burns, observe for CNS symptoms, and to have baselines for follow-up. **I was sent home:** Everything is in slow-motion. I can't think clearly. Even my reflexes are in slow-motion! I can't believe I was sent out to drive forty miles, on a big expressway, in this condition. More unbelievably, I actually made it home. Fortunately, it was two o'clock in the morning. Even now, I try not think about what might have been.

I found that very few of the people I worked with, actually understood the nerve damage that occurs with electrical injuries. I started to look pretty good, on the outside; but inside, symptoms were getting worse. The singed hair I had smelled after the shock, showed up as "spatter" burns on both arms. Seeing another ER doctor to verify the burns: she saw nothing but "dry skin." I asked about the same pattern on both arms? "Yes, that is unusual, I don't know what would have caused that. Try putting lotion on the areas." Again, ignorance was obvious. With a magnifying glass, you could see the small blisters, in various stages of healing; everything from raised reddened pustules, to dimpled and drying water blisters. The red-ear-syndrome (or **RES**, as I would call it) became more prominent. It's difficult hiding the bright red ears. The warmth around the back of the brain was warmer and more bothersome. It felt as if someone was pressing their hand on the back of my head, constantly! What an annoyance! The warmth across my back had become burning. I could not lie on my back. It felt like a terrible sunburn. Once again, the skin looked normal; the damage was underneath. I had surmised that *no feeling* was *good feeling*. Under that burning piece of thick "plastic" that lined my body cavities, I felt nothing. I denied headaches, because "I never have headaches!" With this denial, I used **TOH** for the pain I had on top of the head. After all, it was a pain, not an ache. It made sense to me, at the time. I can call them anything I want, but they may still be termed headaches. My denial had become a choice of ignorance over reality: if I don't see the problem, perhaps it will disappear; like the ostrich hiding his head in the sand. I had this pain about the size of a Ping-Pong ball, in the top of my head; approximately an inch beneath my skull. It was close to the parietal/frontal border, and, while it was hot on the right side, the same area on the left side was just warm and not as intense as the one on the right side of the brain. At times, the pain was so intense, it made my eye squinch and my cheeks would become numb around the eyes. Occasionally, a pain would shoot along a path over the right frontal area, to behind the right eye. Thank Heaven, it never lasted long; 'cause that was some **real pain!** (And yes, after these few years, I still have symptoms. Usually, it is when I am over-tired or have a cold, etc. It seems more prevalent when I am feeling run-down.)

All along, I am like a deer caught in the headlights. I could sense the attitude of "get over it, already." Some even belittled my slow responses; insinuating that I had become senile over-night. They hadn't a clue as to what was going on. My *wrong* words or complete *loss-for-words* became a joke. Fortunately, there were a few, who understood electrical shock; and they worked with me. I am thankful for these few. The others were never too bright about anything they did. We would not expect them to understand. Others would have questions about my peculiar memory deficits. So did I! But, they were curious enough to research the problem. The ignorant believed all present memory was gone, instantaneously. Not so! It's that **20 Minute Delay.** They had learned to take advantage of that delay. I, on the other hand, would become indignant of their behavior, once I had figured out their strategies. It was pretty easy to figure, when I over-heard a couple of the EMTs boasting of how they never did anything, when they were assigned my rooms; "she would just give-up looking for us and do the work by herself," they laughed. It seems, if they played their cards right, they could go a whole night without seeing me. As I entered the "Break Room," they wondered how long I had been standing there. I coyly asked them, "Why, were you talking about me?" They said that they were just talking "guy-talk." Sure! They hadn't realized that I had heard everything. Their lazy shenanigans were recorded, somewhere here. Some things were left in that old computer brain… just not there for voluntary recall. Details slipped away during the night, but that didn't necessarily mean the complete day was missing; just minute details. I would be aware something happened; but, not as to the time or day. Sometimes a *hint* will jar a memory; sometimes it won't mean a thing. It all has to do with the erratic course of the scarred pathway through my brain. I won't really remember much about today, come next week, or the next. Yet, some things are retained and spring back to life, at times when I least expect it; so, that can't be complete amnesia, as many had thought.

Can you believe, these people often tried to take advantage of me, on the premise of my having amnesia? I was especially disappointed at the way the Hospital and their insurance carrier tried to imply that nothing was wrong, and I would be expected to work full-time, when needed. The only details I had retained about my examinations by their doctors was that their doctors had agreed with the findings of my doctors. The Hospital and their insurance representative lied about the doctors reports (some of which they had not yet received.) They must have thought I was nothing but a vegetable. How dare they try something so despicable. Others would take advantage of my memory deficits and the slowed reactions and responses, also.

One day, my head pain had been especially strong, leaving me with even slower reaction time. I signed-up for a lighter work assignment for the day; as others often did "that day of the month," or when they "hadn't slept well the night before," or whatever. We understood. I would take the Urgent Care Rooms. These rooms presented less decision-making problems. The charge nurse of the day stated, "Well, if she wants easy rooms, we'll show her "*easy*." We'll put all of the patients in her beds." She did just that! (Does she think I will forget this? Don't look now, but <u>your</u> ignorance is showing.) I was even given a cardiac patient on a portable monitor, though the two well-equipped cardiac beds across the hall were empty. (That could stack-up well for a law suit against the hospital, if the cardiac patients had problems.) All of the afternoon staff was sitting at the nurses station, making fun of my situation. When I would step out and ask for help, they would say, "Yeah, yeah, just a minute." (Ripe for another law suit!) The doctor who was working with me, finally went looking for help himself, when he would have to stop what he was doing and discharge patients; so he could see the new patients waiting in the waiting room. "What is the matter with you people?! This nurse is overwhelmed with patients, while you sit out here laughing, and doing nothing. And, don't try making excuses, because there is no excuse for your behavior." Their *party* was over; I got my dinner break.

In all walks of life, you will find workers who will only lift a finger, if it's used to pick up their paycheck. Some EMTs were the worse offenders. They could always find a place to hide, if they wanted to get out of work. There were times when you wouldn't see them for the whole shift. (Of course, they had inadvertently, disclosed that little ploy, in the "Break Room.") If they did appear, they would not do the task requested. When I asked one to bathe a patient and get him into a clean gown so the doctor could examine him, I was told, "I cleaned *stuff* when I worked the floors. I don't clean *stuff* any more." (Though his word had been more specific, we'll keep it clean.) When asked who he thought might do it, he replied, "You can do it, when you finish starting that IV." Sure enough, he had disappeared again. Another told me she had never done an enema, and wasn't about to start now. Gee, there were a lot of things in her job description, this girl didn't know how to do. I took her into the room with me, in order to teach her; but, with a nasty look of disgust on her face, she said *she couldn't do it.* It was all she could do, to empty the bedside commode, afterward. I'm sure that the only reason she got this job, was because she knew someone in high places. I have never worked with so many health care workers, with anal phobias. These two had problems emptying a bedpan or a urinal. They even refused to take rectal temperatures on babies. I know, "How sick can you get?" I should have been writing-up all of these weird behaviors, but with my slowed responses, it was too time-consuming. I was being taken advantage of again. Why did they do that?! Because they could. There were very few In Charge, who actually took charge and would over-see the workings of a smooth Unit. Some people are dedicated to their patients, while others are dedicated to themselves, alone. A few nurses would shift their "unwanted patients" into one of my beds, while I was busy… thinking I wouldn't notice? I don't know. I may not remember the details, but I will remember their bizarre problem-solving methods. Not nice! Most workers were considerate and helpful.

A couple of the "Full Time" nurses had even tried to clue-me-in to the fact that the Nurse who did our scheduling was ignoring my request for work. She was using me. She scheduled herself for *doubling-back;* meaning that if she worked more than one shift in one day, she would get paid double-time. She was often too tired to work the sixteen hours, so she would call on we "On-Call" girls to do the extra shift for her. Many times she called me, but I was already working for someone else. She would try to get me to tell the other girl, I couldn't work because I forgot that I was already working for someone else. I told her I would not do that. I would not lie. If I promised to work for someone, they could count on me. My word was good. She cooled to me, real quickly. But, most of the people were a joy to work with. These are the people I will try to remember. (I can always hope, one day my memories will be there, waiting for voluntary recall. You never know!)

Very few of the people I worked with, noticed my personality changes., either. (Or, if they did, they didn't mention it.) Of course, I had only worked at this hospital for a year, when the accident occurred. But, I'm here to tell you, this *prim and proper lady* had had a BIG CHANGE! I had always been reared to believe: An educated person can form a complete sentence without the use of harsh words or slang. So here I am, cussing like a sailor. Birds had always been, "a thing of beauty." Now, I'm *shooting birds* at stupid drivers! My whole adult life, I had felt that arguing was for those at the lower end of the curve, in animal behavior. **Wait.** I am like a child in kindergarten. I just look for things to upset and irritate me; and it wouldn't take much. I even yelled at the "no *stuff* guy," when he again tried to shift a soiled patient into one of my rooms. I told him fine, but he would still need to get the patient ready to be seen by the doctor. He just smirked and said, "That's your problem now; don't call me!" Of course, this was about the time, that his *stuff* hit the fan. The Charge Nurse came to the rescue, when she realized what was happening. His *switch* to get out of work, had been quashed. He WOULD do his job, for a change; but not without his mouthy protest. In order to help the patient bathe and get into a clean gown, he came into the room, looking like someone performing a space walk; face shield, a set of paper scrubs, cap and shoe covers, etc. I would guess that it had been many years since he had truly helped anyone become more comfortable. Obviously, this EMT needed more practice! I'm sure, the spacesuit negated any comfort level. The gentleman just needed someone to bring him a basin of water, some linens and a clean gown. The young man was quite capable of bathing himself. As a lady, I've always said that I might let someone *"walk on me"* occasionally, but don't think you are going to stand there and wipe your feet on me! I'm sure, such a time had come.

What is happening here? You cannot know the embarrassment I felt over these **DECREASED INHIBITIONS;** at least, my neurologist keeps reminding me of this fact. Insisting, "It will get better." "Many people behave this way, all of the time." Of course, she was right; I've seen it time and again, but, that's not ME! Perhaps some thought this to be my normal personality, I don't know; but few detected the difference. (The lazy ones, live for opportunities like this.) I'll admit, you seldom have time for reflections in a busy ER. I think, I had just expected everyone to pick-up-on-it more readily. They were health professionals, after all. The more astute understood the problem, immediately. But, I'm afraid there were few. You can only hope, the astute will be on duty, if any of your friends or relatives are brought in. Either you recognize the symptoms, or you don't. Though symptoms vary, it behooves all workers to know what to look for. Electrical Burns can be serious; AND seriously, hiding beneath a façade of normalcy.

As doctors know very little about electrical trauma burns, why would we expect nurses and other health professionals to understand? My neurologist was amazed, that an ER doctor would discharge a *head trauma victim*, to drive herself home. A victim should be hospitalized for observation. I am sure there has been some enlightenment from her, since then.

The Hospital needed me to see another doctor for their report to the Worker's Compensation Appeals Board. They wanted me to see another one of <u>their</u> neurologist. He would review the case and make sure I received appropriate compensation. **SURE!** Don't we believe that?! The Hospital had sent me to one of their neurologist earlier. He had agreed with my neurologist. (That would be the doctor with the Hospitals' first Insurance Company.) What happened to that doctor?! Now, Workers' Comp would need the opinion of another doctor. Gee, I wonder why. What good would another Workers' Comp Doc do? (It would become very clear to me, many years later.)

This particular doctor, had all of my files to go through, but hadn't realized my appointment was for that day, sooo, he fit me in between his other patients. I had traveled so far to get to his office, in a questionable neighborhood, he didn't dare suggest I come another day. Obviously, this guy had never seen my files before and knew nothing about me, or my condition. He was stuttering so badly, I couldn't concentrate on his questions, or my answers. I could hear him raffling through my files and he would come in and ask a question. Back out to raffle through the files some more, then in for another question. (He must have spent ten minutes, tops, face to face; yet, he charged for an hour and a half.) As he fit me in, I could hear him talking to others, and guess what…NO STUTTERING ! Imagine, a doctor *making fun* of his patient; stuttering, indeed! An astute neurologist would have still been able to have seen what was happening. Since he had not been given a chance to go through my files thoroughly before, he was given another chance to evaluate me; but said that it would not be necessary. **His ignorance was obvious!** (Or, was it pride?) Don't blame him. Most doctors don't really know what to think of Traumatic Electrical Burns. However, one would expect a "***Specialist***" in the field of Neurology to "have an inkling" of what goes on with Electrical Burns. Well, consider this: my brain is still functioning (or malfunctioning) with the same IQ as before, but hasn't the ability to use it as effectively; so, **I am on-to-you!** I just can't do anything about it! Of course, the poor devil decided that I was just playing games. (I should be so lucky as to be able to play any game... Monopoly, Checkers, Go-Fish...any game requiring a little concentration.) Therefore, it was determined I did not rate disability benefits. The Hospital had found **<u>their</u>** ***Preferred Provider!*** Now, who's playing games?

Along with the Worker's Compensation Denial was a form-letter, informing me of the fact that I had the right to get a lawyer and appeal the decision. <u>I am so sure I could have done that!!!</u> I can barely remember what day it is. A stranger on the street could see my disabilities, if he but took the time to talk to me, but this *specialist* found no problems. Yet, my symptoms were so obvious, Social Security wondered why I was not receiving Worker's Compensation. "You should be receiving something every month."

I am not as sharp as I was before the crisis. This Hospital knew exactly what they were doing. Would they feign ignorance as a cover-up? Perhaps, but why would they bother? I couldn't fight a butterfly, in my state of confusion. I refuse to spend the rest of my days fighting a loosing battle. There is no way a big Hospital Conglomerate is going to step-up-to-the-plate and do the right thing. (I would have given them a fight, had I not been mentally challenged.) There is no reason in this world, for a person in my condition, to be expected to give depositions! (Ah, but that's another chapter!) They were aware that I could not assist, on my own behalf. I mean: **Attention Deficit, Short-**

term Memory problems, with **Slowed Responses!** Can you see me, trying to leaf through my daily logs, searching for answers to questions? (Probably forgetting the question, before finding the answer.) I would be of no help. This would have been a real nightmare for my own lawyer, but no lawyer would take my case. Though I had all of the information in writing, I would not be able to assist. As for names, times, dates, and incidents, ***life is a daily occurrence.*** I won't remember my present history; the history after touching that elevator button. I do remember my past history; the history before touching the elevator button. Confusing? You should be in my shoes! I was reminded, time and again, "You can not sue your employer for negligence in California; even continuing negligence!" That is California's **NO-FAULT WORKERS' COMPENSATION LAW**. What kind of **Law** is this, anyway? Somehow, this doesn't sound like a law to protect the Workers' right to compensation, for being hurt on-the-job. It really sounds more like a law to protect the negligent Companies from meeting their responsibilities, under Federal Law. **Who would sponsor such a law?** One can't help wonder if the doctors and lawyers were afraid of losing their reputations (and money), if they went against the State. If so, SHAME ON THEM ALL! And, SHAME ON THE STATE that would hold an injured victim hostage, while intimidating doctors and lawyers to give false reports. At least, that is how I'm seeing things. (Maybe, I just never found a lawyer with guts.) Amazing! But, that's a whole different story! For now, we hope all doctors and medical professionals will put forth an effort to learn about:

THE TRAUMA OF ELECTRICAL BURNS.

Let's educate!

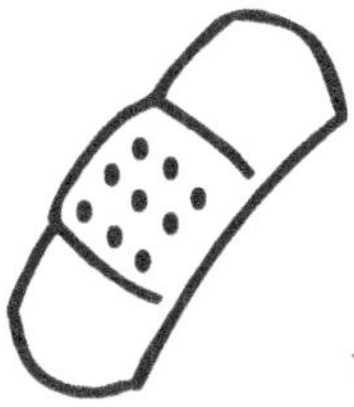

We can hope for compassion and enlightenment,

but, for now, we have to settle for the band-aid.

Sure, we hope to resuscitate their brains, to new horizons.

Still, for many, try as you may, their store is closed, due to

Lack of Stock. And, there is no incoming! Doldrums!

I AM CURIOUS AND I HAVE QUESTIONS!

I'm a little leery; but, is all the world a stage, and we but players? There are so many people playing games, they don't even know they are doing it. Daydreams are supposed to be helpful. I'm not sure we need to be actors, but many do live their lives through the lives of others: in Soap Operas, in Movies, in Sports, in Music, etc. It seems everyone needs to play games. Most games are harmless escapes from the teaming traffic, a rough day at work, or an argument with an acquaintance; a way of clearing your head, so you can think rationally, when over-stressed. Nowadays, when we speak of someone Playing Games, it is usually a negative connotation:

I overhear a doctor trying to recruit other doctors into becoming Expert Witnesses for jury cases. The other doctors said they did not specialize and would not want to alter a case with inadequate information. "Here's the beauty of it all: You don't have to be a specialist, *just a doctor;* that's good enough, and the pay is great!" I didn't see any "takers." That's a relief! You do have better understanding of what goes on in some of these unusual cases, we read about. I know that, if I were on a jury, I would request to see the credentials, which make a doctor a specialist in a particular field. This goes for any *Expert Witness,* no matter what his field.

I've certainly witnessed so much ***"game-playing"*** in the past few months; I could write a book. (But, wait! That's exactly what I'm doing, isn't it?) So, I am more naïve than the average person; still, I expect Health Care Professionals to show more compassion and caring. Let me say, most are genuinely interested in the welfare and good care of each and every patient they see. I'm disgusted with the few who show little or no interest in the patients' concerns or care. I'm aware, every field has its' share of rude, insolent loafers, and manipulators, but you have to blame the ones who permit such behavior. Haven't the doctors noticed the *"Help"* sitting in their office chatting, when there was work to be done? Do Charge Nurses over-look insubordination, because it is easier?

Do Company officials dismiss intolerance and prejudice, by giving preference to the trouble-makers?

Do you remember when over-seas bank accounts were used by spies, to hide their ill-gotten gains? Now, they are used to avoid paying income taxes. Big Corporations used to buy small companies, to pilfer their pension funds. In order to rob pension funds today, the Company makes their employees take Company Stock in place of a pay raise, for their years of faithful work; knowing full-well the stock will be worth pennies, when they take the Company into bankruptcy. So, this is nothing new. Where <u>did</u> we get that saying, *"Going to Hell in a hand-basket"?* (I have an idea.)

Clever Schemes, Hidden Bank Accounts, Creative Bookkeeping, Changing Company Names to cover for Company's misdeeds, Insider Trading, and Golden Parachutes are just a few of the scams out there. Is the behavior of some fellow-workers any different from the above? I think not! They are all, of the same ilk: born Cheaters, Thieves, Manipulators, Rude, Insolent, Inconsiderate, Loafers, M.A.s (not to be confused with M.I.A.s). These people are working hard… to find a place to hide, so they will <u>*miss*</u> any semblance of <u>*action*</u>! Some cannot help themselves. Their lack of conscious is a sociopathic tendency. (Do highfalutin words forgive the sins?) I doubt it. How do we differentiate between harmless games and scams? If no one was hurt by *The Game,* it was harmless. If it hurts others, we have a *Scam*. It is always good to remind ourselves, that

"Your right to swing your fist, stops where my nose begins!"

Let's keep the games clean.

CHAPTER 5

SHOPPING,

A WHOLE NEW WORLD.

SHOPPING . . .
A WHOLE NEW WORLD!

Gosh, where do I begin? There are so many aspects of shopping: groceries, clothes, cleaning supplies, automobiles, houses, plumbing needs, Holiday gifts and cards, linens, furniture, etc. The list goes on. I think you will agree that shopping can be a real challenge anytime. But, for those who are already challenged by the effects of a closed-head injury, it becomes one monumental task. Throw in the **SHORT TERM MEMORY** and **DECREASED INHIBITION,** and you can have a really big problem. If you see something you like, you buy it. Since you really don't remember if you have the same thing at home, you are probably buying duplicates. With that mischievous so-called **20-MINUTE DELAY**, you would buy the item and ask questions later. There is no inhibition to give you a guilty feeling about wasting the money. I guess everyone was pussy-footing around; not wanting to cause any more confusion than I already had. That was appropriate, at the time. What did I know? In this ***FOG***, it was all I could do, to just get through the routine of daily living. I will continue living my life "***one-day-at-a-time***." I sleep and there is a new day, with a new slate. I guess, some would enjoy this predicament, if they could pick their days.

Women everywhere will weep at this sad situation. As I look in my closets, I wonder if I could possibly squeeze in one more item; yet, I haven't a thing to wear. I have clothes that have never been worn; many, still have their price tags. **But, I don't remember what is in my closet from one day to the next!** Just getting dressed, was such an ordeal. I would put on a skirt, then try to find a blouse to match. Now, see if we have earrings to go with this outfit. (If I don't look at home first, I will be buying something to go with it, when I get to the stores.) Are there shoes this color? What sort of purse would work? It took so long to get dressed, because I was constantly running from one closet to another. I can see where one with this condition, might be tempted to lay around in a robe all day; by the time you get dressed, the day is shot! (Especially difficult for one who enjoyed living each moment to the fullest… what a waste of time!) We really do take so much for granted. Getting dressed for work was no problem. I kept my uniforms in one small closet. I could readily see which scrub top went with which scrub pants. Simple! It was the EVERYDAY and DRESS CLOTHES, I found confusing.

If you think it's rough not knowing what you have in the closet, think of your accessories! I do not remember what jewelry I have; what scarves, what purses, what shoes, what jackets, etc. You get the idea! I remember everything I had before I touched the elevator button. It's the purchases I've made and the gifts I've received since, that I don't recall. (And my children wonder why I'm still wearing all of those old-fashioned things! But, these are the things I can remember having; the **B**efore the **C**risis outfits.) I open my jewelry box and **everyday is like Christmas**. I look at my shoes and wonder how I could ever possibly wear them all….and so many the same color! There are many purses…not necessarily matching the shoes; or for that matter, anything else. With the eye of an artist, this perfectionist found it even more difficult choosing an outfit for the day. Only the right shade of a color would do. (I guess that is why I felt a need for blouses in eight shades of purple, fourteen shades of blue to blue-green, six shades of pink, etc.) Gosh! This could be maddening! So, what is the solution?! I wear a lot of jeans and jean shorts….everything goes with jeans. I must admit, I still look for blouses that contain just a speck of steel-gray in the design, or I will wear a solid color. Old habits really do die hard.

Summer is coming and I find the leather tennis shoes heavy and hot. There is new-age material that is light-weight and cool. I must remember to buy some. I was pleased that I could actually remember to look for the light-weight tennis shoes, whenever I passed a display. Just when I thought I was doing better with this *memory thing,* my husband commented on the fact that he thought my new light-weight tennis shoes had blue and green trim instead of the blue and plum trim. I went looking for the blue and green trimmed ones. Found them! Also found the other pair of the blue and plum trimmed ones. **I don't remember buying them!** I pulled out all of my tennis shoes and found that I had twenty pair...... and that doesn't count the five pair of biking shoes.

The shopping problem might have become more obvious, had I not been working the day my husband moved the clothes from one house to the other. Maybe, I could have taken notice and done something about it. I don't know. Like an alcoholic should never drink alone, I should not shop alone. 20/20 Hindsight! I'm told the bed of the pick-up truck was full of my hangered clothes. My husband had missed the opportunity to drive straight to the favorite charity store and unload the clothes there. But, of course, how could he? I was confused enough. He couldn't do that to me.

That's It !!! I am going to give this stuff to charity and start over. My closets are so full, it will take a month to go through everything! Why bother sorting? If I don't remember what is there, I won't miss it anyway. But, should I separate the **BC clothes** from the ones I don't know I have and try wearing my surprise clothes? I'm really not ready for those mysteries, yet.

So, that's not working. I'm still buying things. I see a nice outfit and buy it, without considering all of the excess clothing I already have. I think I need to give up shopping, but that would be depressing. I use shopping as therapy, to get out in the world; it's my contact with others. This way, I don't feel so isolated. We seldom have time to socialize at work. We are lucky to get a supper break, much less a supper break together; it is so busy. If I could just remember not to buy, I'd be in great shape. But, it's as if shopping has become synonymous with buying. I really don't need anything! I have to think of shopping as *WINDOW SHOPPING* or *SIGHT-SEEING.* I am learning! But, slowly.

Every time I think I've made headway, I am reminded that there is no cure for my condition; only, coping. Recently, I felt sure I had bought a certain blouse I had admired. I was going to wear it, but couldn't find it anywhere. To make the hunt more difficult, I couldn't remember if I had decided on the one with the peach background, or the lavender, or the green one. I finally gave up looking. Since I couldn't find it, I must not have bought it, after all. (I probably couldn't decide on a color.) But see, I kind of remember looking at a blouse. To me, that is improvement! I really don't know what sort of design was on the front, but I remembered a blouse from a few days ago. Well, it was just **like Christmas again** when I opened the small suitcase we used for day-trips. There was the Peach Blouse…along with the other things I had forgotten to unpack. Maybe I should check other luggage; but then, if I don't miss it today, I certainly won't miss it tomorrow. Besides I have a bag all ready for travel, on a moments notice.

We went to Florida, for my birthday. It would be good to see my boys. It was the *Rainy Season,* so you never knew when to expect a shower. We came prepared, but my raincoat was so hot and heavy for Florida, I preferred to take my chances. The weather was nice, the first two days; but thunderstorms were predicted, for the next three days. We would be darting in-and-out, looking at houses and sailboats; so, everyone took their raincoats, except me. All of their pleadings, were to no avail. "It would just be too hot." (Of course, I got soaked.) When we arrived home, my husband wondered why I hadn't worn the new micro-fiber coat the boys had bought me the day before. Now, he asks me! (I must have gone to sleep last night.) Of course, I had forgotten it! (Even though, I had worn it the day I received the gift.) That's what we call **short-term memory**. I love that coat! I may have trouble convincing the boys, however.

When I received an invitation to my friends' wedding, I was so excited, I went right out shopping for the *perfect dress*. It was cool out, and wearing a coat is always a hassle when shopping, but I found just the right dress. Happy, I brought it home; and as I hung it in the closet, I wondered, "Whatever would I do with a long-sleeved dress in August?!!! I would burn up!" I kept the dress for other occasions and would shop again for the wedding, come summer. (That so-called **20 Minute Delay** is haunting me!)

It has taken me five years to learn how to shop again! I knew something had to be done, when I would find two of the same design dresses or the same *unique* shorts sets hanging in my closet. You see, my good taste remains: same design dresses, but in two different colors. Again, I had bought this nice shorts outfit, while vacationing in Florida. It was in shades of blue and aqua (favorite colors), with a seashell motif (appealing to a scuba diver). I brought it home and hung it in the closet… right next to an identical set, I must have purchased before going on vacation. Wow! What that does to your self-esteem! Well, no one would know but me. Eventually, I would come to realize that I did not have to BUY, when I went WINDOW SHOPPING. I could relax and meander through the mall, at my leisure. I am no longer rushing around, trying to find something to buy. I had finally learned to truly enjoy a day of window shopping; without buying. I can still enjoy the laughter and the stimulating interaction with others. When I really need something for a special occasion? I shop at home. In my closets are pre-selected items of my choosing, in the right size and colors; all I have to do, is sort them out. This gives a whole new meaning to "Home Shopping," doesn't it? Well, it works for me.

Clothing was not the only problem. It was just an example of my many problems. Another might be the "tree." I was at a nursery and spotted a rare tree, with which my son had always been fascinated. He was going to get a place of his own and that would make such a nice house-warming gift. He would love it. I paid for the tree but would have to come back, with a van or truck, to transport it home. When my son came home from work, I told him of the prize I had found. He said that, while it was a great gesture; he hadn't even decided on whether he would be buying a house, a town house, or a condo. We both knew that I had had another problem with my **"Lag Time."** Not to worry. We just went back to the nursery and received a refund.

* * * * * * *

My husband must have a multitude of "stars in his crown!" What a saint! We went shopping for a car. Every man enjoys that little shopping spree -- (though, they hate shopping for anything else.) We test-drove several models, before we decided on the one to buy. However, months from now, I will still be looking for features that were in other models. I could have sworn this car did not have a passenger-side airbag. "Your old car didn't, but this one does." The sun's in my eyes - we'll just pull over those visor extensions. "No, that was in another model we drove." As we approach the toll plaza, I'm looking for the money in my little cubbyhole. "That was the old car." These are lousy cup-holders! Why did we buy a new car, anyway? I'm reminded of the safety features AND the fact that I needed a car to "fit me." A tilt wheel that brings the wheel close enough that it won't strain my *tennis elbows* or the *injured shoulders.* One with a seat that would adjust to ease *arthritic hips.* Oh, now I remember. I used to have a lot of pain driving long trips. Driving is much more pleasant, since we bought this car.

So, for you younger ones, who wonder about all of those old folks driving big cars they can barely handle, I'm divulging the answer: Those are the cars with the softer rides over the railroad tracks, well-cushioned seats, automatic everything, more room for walkers and wheelchairs, and wider carriage space. (Spacious seats, for spacious seats.) Also, safer for occupants of diminishing eyesight, who play a lot of *Bumper Cars.* Everyone will be able to see the PAPA DOC's in time to avoid them, when they are driving bigger cars. I have coined this phrase to describe little old dictators ... you know the ones: They enter the expressway doing 35mph (I know the Sixteen-wheelers love these people. That is a lot of steel to bring to a stop, when you are trucking at 55mph!); or, they drive 55mph in the fast lane, even though the speed limit is 65mph, 'cause "No one needs to be driving faster than 55mph" (for my father, it had been 45mph); or, they set their fancy new cruise control to 60mph. I mean, how can one be sure the cruise control is accurate? They don't want to be caught speeding. (People of that generation, often distrust *new technology.*) Then, they stay in the fast lane with their right blinker on; because they will be driving through for the next seven miles, <u>but</u> want the other cars to know that they will be getting off soon. (And, haven't we all zipped around them, by then?) We know that these *careful drivers* usually drive certain makes of cars...don't follow them! (Besides, some are still looking for their lost cubbyholes.)

An FYI **Observation and Road Report** from a non-challenged driver! Rush Hour Traffic tells us that many drivers are mentally challenged. There is the "get out of the way" Road Rage. What has happened to common courtesy?

I'm afraid it has disappeared, along with common sense. Should we even mention the thousands of mentally deficient drivers, who don't know the difference between YIELD and MERGE? Where did they learn to drive? A refresher: ***Yield*** means you cautiously approach an intersection and give way to the car with the right-of-way. ***Merge*** means that you build-up to expressway speed before entering the expressway. That is why we have merge lanes, and that is why the on-going traffic would, *usually*, move to the left; speed-up to allow a slower auto to meld-in; or, slow a bit, to "fall-in" behind the faster vehicle, to allow the merge. Reality Check! We are not sitting at a stop sign, waiting for a break in traffic. We have increased our speed, in order to merge. Can you tell me where we are supposed to go, at 55-65mph, when the merge lane ends? (Watch your language!)

Like I say, there are many challenged drivers. I really don't think cell phones have helped driving performance, either. I can see that I am not the only one in this world, who cannot handle more than one task at a time. It's sort of like the old saying, "He can't walk and chew gum at the same time." This is the person who should not have a cell phone in his hand, while driving. Do you realize that hands-free devises do little to conquer distraction? It seems that the attention you need to carry on a conversation, is a huge distraction, in itself. When statistics tell us that one in four accidents are caused by distractions, it's time we pay attention. All of these distractions, make us the equivalent of *a drunk driver*. (Ah, but you good church-going people don't even drink.) My son had his car totaled, while sitting at a stop light. He was hit from behind, by a driver on a cell phone, who had not even slowed for the light. No, he wasn't a drunk driver; just a distracted driver. Seriously, considering the danger, is there ever time so pressing, when you could not wait until you park the car, before using a cell phone, eating a snack, changing the CD, adjusting your seat, or *adjusting* the kids in the back seat? Maybe, we need to check our own behavior, while being aware of the other distracted drivers out there. Driving is a full-time job. I was amazed and very relieved to learn that my driving remained as crisp and reactive as it had been before the SHOCK. That's a blessing! God knows, you have to be ever vigilant, with today's driving conditions. I think that courteous driving comes naturally; an extension of oneself. You can tell a lot about a person, by the way they drive.

* * * * * * *

A woman's work is never done; especially, when she does everything twice! Grocery Shopping is every woman's bane. Just try buying the items for a menu, when you don't know where they are kept in the store. The overhead departmental signs help, but not much. (I am so *totally* lost, in a strange store.) I never realized, I cooked with so many specialty items, until this thing happened. Does it really matter? I bring the groceries home and put them away and (are you following this?) ….I don't remember why I bought the cabbage. It is not St. Patrick's Day! Cole slaw is always good. We rarely have that. So, when I notice green peppers in the crisper that are getting long-in-tooth, I remember that I had planned on making stuffed cabbages. (Yes, we like them with green peppers and onions seasoning them.) So, groceries are another example of *"Out of sight, out of mind."* If you think that's tough, try finding the things in your own kitchen, after a two-week vacation. I've learned to watch my husband, to see where he goes for his cereal, bowl, and spoon. I do get used to my routine again, in a day or two. See, whenever I start feeling better about my abilities, something like this slaps me back to the reality, that there really are permanent disabilities! Some of us will be working over-time to convince others that we have no problems. We are too proud to settle for less than the best. If I can learn to accept, then I will learn to adapt, instead of playing a "cover-up" game.

Supermarket Specials are always appreciated. Since we like everything and will eat anything; whatever is on sale for the week, is on the menu. The only problem I have with this is … I glance at the ad before going to the store, write a list, and buy the specials. (Those darn ads can run a week or two.) How many times do I need to buy the same specials? I don't know. Check my cupboards, frig, and freezer. I could feed an army for a year! It comes in handy, when the budget is tight for a week or two. (Of course, the budget probably wouldn't be so tight, if I wasn't buying duplicate groceries!) Fortunately, I've always been a proficient cook. You know, never two meat loaves the same. Usually, whatever I find in the frig or pantry becomes dinner. Sort of like going on a scavenger hunt. I am so thankful that my family will eat anything you put before them. Perhaps, a learned necessity of frugal living. Nobody can do magic with ground beef, like a Serviceman's Wife; or the Single Girls, fresh out of school. I've cooked all of the usual dishes, plus a few unusual ones, I've made-up along the way. Have any of you girls forgotten the time we pooled our money and bought a half of a pound of hamburger, to go with the package of macaroni, half of a green pepper, an onion, and small can of tomatoes? I know that memory has to be right up there, next to the tuna casserole and red wine. (Our paychecks went for the latest styles and other necessities: like rent and utilities.) I can barely tolerate grilled cheese sandwiches, to this day. They tell us, all of those perplexing experiences in our lives, teach us to handle the obstacles in our future. I must agree.

I smile, as I journey back in thought (**B**efore the **C**risis), to when my children were young. I had gotten a recipe out of the newspaper for "Angel Rolls." I'm thinking, these things must be real miracles! They don't even require yeast! I was curious, and had to try them for dinner. (I was so young and gullible.) All of that work, and they were like hockey pucks! We were too poor to waste all of those ingredients, so we had "English Scones" for dinner. No one was the wiser. The older boy even had something to talk about in his geography class. "In England, they eat scones. My mother made some for us, last night for dinner." That was well and good until Parent/Teachers night. His teacher thought that I was such a great parent. True, we did try to teach interesting bits to our children. (I didn't have the heart to tell my boys that the paper corrected it's mistake the next day…we were to add a cake of yeast. SOME MIRACLE! And, hadn't my Mother taught me to *believe nothing you hear, and only half of what you see*?) Well, the teacher and I had a good laugh. Besides, they did taste a lot like scones; even if the texture was more like stones. I mean, could you ask for a better family?

My meals are always a wonder, now. I wonder what I can do with this and a can of soup….(never mind what recipe I had in mind, when I bought it; those ideas died over-night, with the rest of my **Short-term Memory.**). There is still another problem. I generally fix two types of meat loaves: a sweet and spicy Bahamian meat loaf, if it is going to be used for dinner; or a hot and spicy one, if we are going to use it for sandwiches. Generally, they are *general;* but throw in a computer glitch, and the simple meat loaf becomes *frustration*! I was fixing a hot and spicy number, but I couldn't remember what I used for "hot." I kept adding different spices; cumin, red pepper, Cajun spice, hot sauce, etc. Still, I felt something was missing. With the unfamiliar smell coming from the oven, the dropped information returned. Of course, CHILI POWDER! It was as if I had never heard of this wonderful spice. While I hate computer glitches, **glitches from the brain** are worse. Adding the other spices and extra garlic, did not take the place of the chili powder! For some things, there are no substitutes.

A recent Thanksgiving morning, I wanted to make my husband's favorite Cranberry/Apple Bake. The cranberries had to be chopped, but my portable chopper had lost its ability to hold a charge. (Rechargeable appliances are convenient, but they don't usually last long.) I had put the turkey in the oven and sit down to slice the cranberries in two, when my husband asked if there was anything he could do. "Sure, grab a knife and help me slice these cranberries." "Why aren't you using your food chopper?" he asked. I reminded him that its battery had gone bad. "That was years ago!" He continued, "We bought an immediate replacement. It is electric, not battery operated. You used it to chop vegetables for soup last winter." (That's news to me. I don't know anything about an electric chopper.) "Well, if I have one, where is it?" He said he would find it for me. AND, HE DID! I just wonder how many times I've worked-my-fingers-to-the-bones, slicing and dicing vegetables, when I could have saved time and aggravation with my fancy chopper. Oh, well. Another dropped chip! I did recognize it and knew how to work it, once I saw it again. In order to cope with these faulty chips, I plan to have one of those roll-top cupboards in the corner of my next kitchen. I can store all of my appliances in one spot, so I can see what I possess. Perhaps, it would be wise to label all of my kitchen cabinets and drawers, also. Whether I like it or not, everyday will always be a brand new adventure, with no help from the day before. What can I say?

I'm doing so much better, now. I can laugh at my surprise meals. This was my greatest asset, in overcoming, or accepting, many of my disabilities. When this SHOCK first happened, it was not the least bit funny! I had thought that I could go right on cooking, the way I always had; not so! I learned that all of these things that had become a part of me, were no longer within my control. I knew how to use the stove and microwave; just, not how to assemble the ingredients. The first time I made *Chicken a la orange* (a staple in my repertoire), I could not identify the finished product. I knew it was chicken breasts, but I had left out so many ingredients, it actually tasted like chicken breasts! No ginger. No onions. No brown sugar. **I was crushed!** (I blamed that darn **Attention Deficit!**) I had all of the ingredients ready; but, I was so involved, trying to make the fried rice, while cooking the chicken, I just forgot to put them in. **How would I ever cook again?!** (By repetition, that's how!) I learned to start simple. I will always have problems with too much detail. I can only concentrate on one dish at a time. (If I am intent on making a specific dish, I will have to resort to using a recipe.) Do you want to know what is really embarrassing? It's when someone asks me for the recipe for that *great pasta salad* I brought to the covered dish supper; what can I say? "I don't remember what I put in it." Sure! They think you are just trying to guard your recipe. I'm Not! Like my meat loaves, never two salads the same. **I** can't even repeat the same recipe. Forget the repertoire. (I have!) Just wing-it. Whatever spices I think will go with a particular meat, vegetable, or pasta; it becomes dinner. Cast a few spices around, and everything taste gourmet. (Barring, computer glitches!) No English Scones lately, but I have seen a few fallen cakes and dry lasagna. Crumble the cake into pudding or over ice cream for a "different" dessert. The lasagna can be saved by adding a cup of cottage cheese and warming it in the microwave. (Very Moist!) The secret of a proficient cook is to see *what you have wrought before you* and then, looking around to see what you can use for a "save." If you haven't the time and the lasagna is dry, you can always end the meal with a <u>different</u> dessert.

* * * * * * *

It was obvious, from the time of the SHOCK, that I was having some real difficulties getting my brain and hands working together. I immediately started using my husbands computer mouse, in hopes of helping my hand/eye coordination. Even though the doctors said that P.T. wouldn't help, I had to feel that I was trying something; anything that might retrain my scarred pathways. I knew I could not master a computer, but with the help of my husband, I learned to play Solitaire. I wish I could say that the games brought about miraculous improvements, but the right hand is still slower than the left and getting the hands to do what I want them to do, is still impossible. (As I proofed my book, I'm realizing ten years later, that it is the left hand instead of the right hand, that is slower. Or maybe, I'm ambidextrous, where this is concerned.) The one thing the computer game did for me, was to check the speed of my responses to stimuli. If I could play a game of Solitaire without problems, it would be a good day to tackle other things. If I had difficulty with Solitaire, stay away from new challenges for the day.

Still in denial, another big-time problem I had not anticipated, was the *Patterned Potential for Disaster.* I had always designed and sewn my own clothes; plus, making "matching shirts" for my husband and my two boys. Now, I wanted to make a couple of weskits, so I bought a pattern. (Normally, patterns were not necessary for me.) I understood that I was having the eye/hand coordination problem, so I figured a pattern would make things easier. **I am so wrong!!!** Can you imagine my amazement?!! I cut out the pattern pieces and lay them on the table. It was as if someone had thrown a 2000-piece puzzle on the table, without a picture, and told me to put it together. Nothing made sense. My brain knows how these things go together, logically; but my hands are confused as to how to carry out the task. (I understand that this is just an example of my **MOTOR APRAXIA**. And, I suppose the apraxia is why I keep putting my pull-over shirts and sweaters on backwards.) Well, those were weskits; pretty involved. Yet, I found myself in the same predicament, when trying to make simple pillowcases. If I make the mistake, I can see how to correct it; still, my hands won't cooperate. For a pillowcase, I will try; for anything else, I will buy. I was sorry I had bought all of that material for those custom-made pillows, I had planned to sew for my sons' Christmas gifts. Don't hold your breath, guys. Believe me, they wouldn't look that great, anyhow. (I've got a puzzle, I might send you. Hint: It is supposed to be a weskit.)

Of course, I never say never. What nobody else can do, I can. After all, I was in a *fog* for six long years, but that has cleared. It will be different, this time. We bought a sail cover for the boat. Very expensive! I could have made it for half the price. **I will** make the cover for the jib sail. That should be a snap. Just in case, I'm taking no chances. We borrowed a friends jib cover and traced a pattern. So far, so good. I explained to my husband about the material having a "right" side and a "wrong" side. Even though both sides looked the same, they weren't. We lay the material down and put the pattern on top of it. WAIT! We have plenty of length, but the material is not wide enough. WHAT WAS I THINKING? How can we cut two of these curved pieces from the one width of material? (Have I said how glad I am that my husband is an aircraft A&P and a machinist?) He could immediately see, how it had to be done…unfold the material, flip the pattern around; then the narrow part of the pattern will be over the wide part of the material, you just cut out. (Yeah, that's the ticket! And what I had planned, when I bought the material!) I flipped the pattern and was ready to cut, when the machinist had to convince me that we would have to turn the material over (on the "wrong" side) while using the wrong side of the pattern, if we were going to insure that the "right" sides were right. (Of course, I know that, but my hand/eye coordination is still off. Not to mention, the silly **20-MINUTE DELAY** in my assimilation/reaction time.) I'm not totally sure he has convinced me of anything. I know the project came out alright; but, every time we go over the procedure, none of it makes sense! I really hate admitting defeat. I could not have accomplished this task, without my husband. If someone puts the pieces of the puzzle together, I can still run the sewing machine. BIG DEAL! So, it may take a little more time to overcome this obstacle. **More denial!** I think I need to accept my limits. It seems there are many. Maybe saving money is not so important as saving peace-of-mind.

There are a lot of things I did before, taken for granted, I cannot do now. Just one of those things might be the enjoyment of picking out the right birthday card. Usually, one would go to the card store and buy cards for any occasion coming up, within the next three months. This is preferable to going shopping every month. It's often difficult finding the time to do so, and I like being prepared. Remember, I forget! I will be shopping for a card again, closer to the date; just as well, I don't remember where I stored the others. I come across them, at one time or another, in some file folder or drawer .... Oh well, I'm prepared for next year. (Wanna bet?) Still, I manage to send the card too late or too early. My father-in-law received his last card five weeks early. Since my husband and his birthday are four days apart, I certainly knew the date of his birthday; yet, my father-in-law felt the need to remind me of his *correct* birth date, when he thanked me for the card. I guess he forgets that I forget. What a pair we make!

My sons have birthdays three days apart. They will often get the same card – and gift. The older one will ask the younger one what they had received for their birthday, before he opens his gift. I really have to shop and ship at the same time. I'm learning, but it took a long time. As before the near-electrocution, I would buy Christmas Gifts and hide them in different little places, until I got them all together for wrapping and giving. (I will find them eventually, but it is not as if you can give the fur-lined leather gloves for an August birthday.) I coped by wrapping and tagging the gifts as soon as I bought them. That sounds like a good solution! I can beat this problem! Well, not quite. If I wrap them ahead of time, I might have to open them again to see what I had bought, so I wouldn't buy the same thing twice. Finally, I've learned to *wrap*, *tag*, and *identify* the contents on the back of the tag in Gregg shorthand. (I know they won't figure this out; none of them have taken Gregg shorthand. Besides, I have a hard enough time figuring it out myself.) No more repeat gifts! (Unless it's a year or two later.)

My mind tells me I can do anything I did before the incident, but I really can't. I can remember everything that happened before the incident, so why can't I do these things? Obviously, I knew how to do them before; why not now? I can still drive a car, so why can't I sew? (I will always have questions, with no answers.) A confusing mystery! It's that darn delay in assimilation and logical thinking that prevents many of my tasks. Perhaps sewing requires constant assimilation of new information and more intense thought processes than Attention Deficit will allow. (Or, might it just be the Rouge Roads, again? That tangle of scarred pathways, sending confusing signals.) See, I am still telling myself that all of these things, which once came so easily, are a snap. **BIG TIME DENIAL**. I know that the eye/hand coordination is no longer working correctly. Nine years later, that has not changed! Do you know how difficult it is to draw a simple diagram? When I chipped my right front tooth, I could not make a diagram of it, because of the eye/hand problem. I had two teeth in the diagram, but which one depicted the right tooth? I don't know! And, this is nine years later?! I still hold out hope for more recovery, despite the caution of all of the doctors. They could be wrong. But then, this is just another obstacle, I choose to ignore. ***COTTON PICKIN' COCK-EYED OPTIMIST!*** I think that, given time, I can overcome this problem. (Of course, that won't happen.) Like my other obstacles, I will learn to live again, when I learn to **live with *what has become permanent***.

CHAPTER 6

FAULTY

NERVE ENDINGS

FAULTY NERVE ENDINGS.

I was on my stationary bike one morning, when my husband walked into the room and said, "Guess what you forgot!" I gave him the blank look, so he continued with a few hints… "The bananas. Last night." Yes. (If you buy a large quantity of bananas and want to retard the ripening, you just put them into the refrigerator for twenty minutes and it will stop the process.) I had put them in, while getting ready for bed the night before. My husband had asked if I was sure I wouldn't forget to take them out before going to bed. I assured him that I would not forget. (Bless his heart; he still has so much faith in my ability.) Now, we burst into laughter. I can't even remember what I am supposed to remember, much less what I'm not supposed to forget!! I will experience my so-called **"20 MINUTE DELAY"** and the frustrating "**MEMORY GLITCHES"** for the rest of my life. (I think I am past the feeling of embarrassment.) I'm learning to live with them. There was once a comedian who had an act, where he used like-words in his sentences, but they made the meanings completely different. I could have the same act. I know the right word, but it doesn't always come out. You know, *instigate* instead of *initiate,* or *mediaeval* instead of *medial*. Worse yet: "My words escape me." or "I'm at a complete loss for words." "No. Really. I am at a complete loss for words." Right in the middle of a sentence, there is *no word*…a complete computer shutdown. I will rack-my-brain for months sometimes, before a word returns. (Never more evident, than while writing this book. I had to make it a game of *fill-in-the-blanks* later, or I would never have finished.)

It has taken a long time to get to this point… where I can laugh at myself. Believe me, I found nothing funny about imperfection. As a frustrated perfectionist, I was willing to overlook imperfection in others, but set impossible goals for myself. Yet, I think this is how I have accomplished many things in my life. There will always be many trials and tribulations to overcome, but many more triumphs and joys along the way, also. We will focus on the positive.

I am **RE-LEARNING TO "PLAY THE GAME."** My personality was wiped-out in a split second. I am learning social graces all over again. The neurologist told me that, after four years, I had regained all I could expect to regain. I am, what I am going to be, and I would have to learn to live with it. On the way home, I had never felt so lonely in my life. What good is life, like this? As long as there was hope of getting over this, I was willing to fight, but, now.... I don't know. Am I strong enough to accept this?! (Just part of the decreased inhibitions; I had never doubted my abilities before, so why now?) What do you do in a situation like this? I looked up and called out, "God, what is wrong with me? I've never been like this. I'm not ME." Just as quickly, the answer came: of course, I'm not me; I've had a brain injury. Through my tears, I heard a new song come on my car radio. It was a song of encouragement; how you've handled many obstacles in your life, and you can certainly handle this. It was precisely what I needed to hear, at that exact time. I wonder if these artists know how therapeutic their music can be, or just how much good they do. (Laugh, and the world laughs with you. Cry, and you cry alone.) That day, I chose to laugh again. I will get on with my life. And, I will enjoy!

I am no longer flipping birds at rude drivers, or swearing like a sailor. I have gotten over the *childish behavior, delicate feelings, arguing,* and ... oh yes, the innocence of saying whatever comes to mind without thinking of the consequences. MY! MY! MY! What's so bad about that? My words might have been different, had I taken 20-30 minutes to consider the variables. Didn't our mothers teach us not to say anything, if we couldn't say something nice?

(In short, I'm learning to keep my mouth shut!) Would you tell an acquaintance that her hair looked better long? I don't think so … she can't glue it back. Don't we all know better than to get into the middle of a lovers' quarrel? "He's a rat and doesn't deserve you. You can do so much better." You know, as soon as you say something like that, there will be a wedding … and you are not invited! "What's wrong with your nose?!" (It's a big red pimple. Thanks for pointing it out.) How about, "Your shirt is wrong-side-out." "Did you know your socks are different colors?" "What's wrong with your face? Did you cut yourself shaving? Oh no. I see you just forgot to remove the acne cream." Being so darn helpful could get you a punch in the nose. Let someone else play the fall-guy… I'm saying nothing.

I'm learning sleight-of-hand (or should I say, sleight-of-lips?) I often have a loss for words right in the middle of a sentence. I've learned to just change the subject real quick. Everyone has a loss for words occasionally, but you could always find a few synonyms to substitute and no one was the wiser. It's not like that now. *It's like my computer has a faulty chip and has dropped the information completely.* My friends and family realize, when I call a squirrel a cat or a windmill a lawnmower, I really do know the difference. When I have that "loss for words," they have permission to fill in the blanks; even if sometimes, it seems we're playing *"Twenty Questions."* They have gotten used to me.

LAG-TIME will forever haunt me! This is where the brain is slow to assimilate information and turn it around with the appropriate reflex or response. It takes about twenty minutes for it to catch up; or longer. I may answer a question one way, then after the usual "ifs" "ands" and "buts," the answer would be completely different. (i.e.) My doctor sends me to a specialist for an EMG of the ears to check out a persistant episode of dizziness. The specialist asked if my sinuses are bothering me. I told him "NO." On the way home, I beat myself to death because I answered him as if he had asked "Are your sinuses bothering you right now?" I've had Chronic Sinusitis for years, but he'll never know! A new doctor may ask me to tell him about my current medications and what I use them for. Bad move! I may not get past number one, after describing what I use it for. With the attention deficit, they may want to prod me on a bit… "Anything else?" I will make an appointment to see my doctor, but by the time I get in to see him, I will have forgotten what I was there for. (The two days of chest pain were obviously nothing serious … I'm still here.) My regular doctors wonder why I have a list of symptoms or questions with me. You see that look of wonder… "Why is she pulling out a piece of paper? Doesn't she remember anything? Oh yeah…she doesn't!" LISTS are a great help, **IF** you remember to take them out of your pocket.

Perhaps, my doctors should keep me waiting, after they have seen me. This would give me time to assimilate the information received. The Doc could then give me a pop quiz, to make sure I had comprehended his instructions. Focusing on the subject for a while, may clarify matters. Then again, it may not. Besides, the longer one lingers in a doctor's waiting room, the more one becomes exposed. No, I'm not speaking of diseases. I'm speaking of exposure to nosy people. Will they notice the bright red ears (or, The Red Ear Syndrome, as I call them.)? They will appear, even to this day. Sometimes I can wear earrings, sometimes, I can't. Most strangers would make a passing comment about my sunburned ears and wonder how I managed to burn *just the ears.* I could tell them that they are not really sunburned, but just feel and look sunburned. I could go into the "wrong message being sent by the brain," but I don't. I usually just smile and shrug my shoulders. (Actually, they feel like a big mosquito bite.) Yet, the most fun I could make of this situation, was the child I had in Triage. Kids will say anything… "Look Mommy. Her ears are like Rudolph's nose." It was the Christmas Season. I hadn't been able to describe them before. Now, I can.

Will people notice the long pause, as I go from one mode to another? Like your digital watch: you can set the hour, but will have to change modes, in order to set the minutes. If I am deep into reading a magazine article and you ask me to pass you a magazine, I will be at a loss for words for a few seconds. I must change from the reading mode, of interaction with an inanimate object; to the reality mode, of interacting with a human subject. (Usually, courtesy dictates you exchange verbal pleasantries, while passing the magazine.) Of course, they are going to notice!

I will always go home with the questions I forgot to ask; and **forget about ever talking to a doctor by phone**, when I do remember the question. They are too swamped. You could wait for hours, till they return your call. (By then, I will have forgotten the question anyway.... Unless I remembered to write it down... Not Likely!) I cannot tell you how many things have been left unsaid. "Remind your doctor..." "Let your husband know..." "Be sure to try ..." "Its on sale at ..." "Don't forget to come 30 minutes early..." "Send me the information..." Yeah, sure! Please! Write it down, doc. Remind me again the day of the party or the dental appointment. I'm sorry it has come to this, but it is a part of my getting-on-with-my-life. Thanks.

Since my circuitry is so screwed-up, why must I be able to feel things erratically? I mean, I wish I could choose my poison. I would not have chosen to feel the HIVES (Urticaria) that became a daily occurrence in their six months existence. They had been intermittent, for the first four months, then, daily. There never seemed to be a causal relationship... no rhyme or reason. I might have one on my right heel, one on my left thigh, one on the back of my head, and one on my eyelid, all at once. Rarely the same place twice. Like the other phenomena, nothing made sense to me. (To the doctor, it was to be expected. The brain was sending false messages. After all, the nerve pathways had suffered traumatic burns. We should expect the unexpected.) I speak from the voice of much experience; the very worse place for a hive is **on the top of your foot, under your shoestrings, while driving a busy expressway!!** (Having hives on the bottom of your feet would come in at a close second.) There is no way you can rub it gently with your other shoe. You cannot apply a soothing lotion. You cannot scratch it vigorously with your nails. You have to grit your teeth and hold everything in. This was so nerve-wracking! At work, I could take care of my patients, but I was anxiously awaiting the opportunity to dash into the ladies room, loosen my clothes, apply the cortisone cream to air-dry, before tightening my clothes and going back to work. If you were to look in the dictionary, this would be the description of *EXTREME STRESS!*

The most notable hive experience, had to be the two big hives running down the outside of each leg. They were solid welts, about an inch and a quarter wide, and running from the hips to three inches below the knees. It was as if some joker had put a yardstick against my legs and had drawn these welts. Again, no rhyme or reason for them… I was wearing loose shorts and seamless panties. Perhaps, I had been Napoleon in another life; or a football player from the past. The "stripes" were like the pattern on a uniform. The welts were raised and the edges clean as a pencil line. (I suppose, I can accept that these were not merely hives, but angioneurotic edema.) As cute and interesting as they were, they still itched like the devil. Despite all treatment, they remained for two hours.

My hives will have persisted, with some frequency, the first two years. We had tried everything, or so I thought. My doctor sent me to an allergist. He put me on Seldane, AND THE HIVES WERE GONE!!! I could not believe the relief I received from that day on! It had all been a fishing trip, but finally paid off. Everyone is different. What works for one, may not work for another. Remember, all medication has side-affects. I occasionally get hives today, but half a pill works fine. (Of course, I begin to notice an irregular pulse, after the occasional half pill. The Cardiologist pulled that pill immediately. Like they say, medicine is not an exact science. There is a lot of trial and error, before they find what is right for you. And, what is right for one problem, may not be right for other conditions, you may have. Keep all of your doctors apprised of your current medications.)

You hear talk of *raw nerves.* I think I know what they mean: Keeping silent, when you wanted to scream. (I did go through a lot of *Silent Screams!*) Gritting your teeth, when you knew it would just wear them down. Refraining, when you wanted to claw yourself. Controlling the urge to rip your clothes off. **Think of this mental anguish!!** It took such discipline! I'm sure I'm a much calmer person today. I can afford to be, with the hives relieved. BUT, during those times of constant itching, I was one heck-of-a-mess! This is all a viscous circle: Confusion heaped on confusion of symptoms; symptoms causing confusion. There is the Slow Motion, the Fog, Pressure on the back of my head, Numb Cheeks, Head Pain, Hives, "Sunburn," etc.; just to mention a few. Just how does one function, in this condition? With an unbridled stubborn self-determination, that's how.

Then, this inability to sense HOT or COLD was just another aggravation. My husband came home from work one summers night to find the windows fogged-up. With the air conditioner on, the temperature had gone down to 65 degrees! Since I don't feel temperature on my skin or get goose flesh, I had no idea. Had it been daylight, I would have seen the fogged windows. I put my hand on my legs, and could sense I should be cold. I should have goose bumps. That was strange; I could feel that my skin was cool, by the touch of my palms. It would seem I should be able to sense it from the brain. ("The brain is sending false messages, again." No need to mention the malfunction of the hypothalamus, because everything is malfunctioning.)

On winter nights, as we left work, we could see our breaths and be scraping ice off our car windows; I would be comfortable in shirtsleeves, while everyone else was wearing heavy coats. I went through several winters this way. Strangers were commenting on the fact that I was wearing jeans shorts instead of jeans. Wasn't I cold? No, I was comfortable. I would reason: Maybe the same temperature in Florida seemed colder, with the high humidity. I had lived there for thirty-six years. (It would be six more winters before I ever felt cold again and had to wear long pants and a coat.) I do have to be very careful of those *warm* relaxing baths. Invariably, the water is too hot, but I don't feel it. If I step in and can see a red demarcation line, I know to step out and add cold water. I really should use a thermometer. I may never sense hot and cold as normal people do. Still, I'm making progress.

I don't perspire as much as others, either. There were only two times this proved embarrassing. We attended an Air Show on a hot summers day. I must have gotten over-heated. As I walked into the air-conditioned house, I found myself with a mouth-full of emesis. (Fortunately, there was a bathroom next to the entry.) **I don't feel peristalsis, so why would I feel reverse peristalsis?!** This would happen again, while hiking, leaving a restaurant, and during a bout with the flu. It was tense! As a pilot must always have an alternate landing spot in mind, I had to be constantly aware of where I could go, in an emergency. (Those plastic-lined wastebaskets would be my savior, at work.) I wish I could be sure I would never have trouble with reverse peristalsis again, but eight years later I awakened with a mouth-full of emesis. (It's a good thing I sleep on my side.) Is it any wonder I refuse sleeping pills and other depressants?! I certainly don't need to depress my functions.

Within those first few months, there was this other little problem…Not being able to feel intestinal movements or cramping, I would pass gas with the reverberation of the boys in a third grade class. The innocent looking nurse seemed crass. A lady would *feel a song coming on* and seek the restroom. A couple of guys at work would say, "There she goes, she's farting-around again." They had fun. What could I say? I was! This situation would humble the most confident lady. Especially embarrassing was hearing my walking cadence. I do walk fast. I learned to slow down.

This was not supposed to happen. Even my own doctor suggested my not telling anyone about the next subject... "Doctors don't understand. Certainly, the average person is not going to understand, what makes these things happen." (If you find gross reality a problem, skip the next three paragraphs.) Since this book is for enlightenment, I must tell about my experiences. I feel compelled to write about this subject, for the patients who are not nurses. Perhaps we can avoid needless intestinal blocks. (Perforation is often a consequence of Electrical Injury.) We don't want to dwell on the situation, but need to be aware that some nerves have been damaged, and they may disrupt any of the *bodily functions*.

As I spoke of the wrong messages being sent by the brain, this also was a part of the wrong messages being sent. That first year, on two different occasions, I would experience colon aperistalsis. I'm reminded of that white wood glue on the back of the workbench. If you leave the cap off, you will find a hardened plug of glue you must remove before you can get to the soft part. On those occasions, I would find the bottle of glue full, but unable to expel it. There was no hardened plug; the stool was just there! Fortunately, the sphincter was working! There was no peristalsis. (Believe me when I say, if you had been eating oatmeal everyday for years, you would be assured of a stool of perfect consistency, which was easily evacuated.) Usually, in a day or two, I would have to remove a drying plug and do a digital evacuation of the soft stool; something a nurse is proficient doing. (However, a contortionist would have been more suited for this job; since it was being performed by the other end, of the same person. But, that's a horse of a different color.) There was no problem, other than the colon's inability to contract those circular muscles needed for peristalsis; to move things along the tract. The peristalic wave was in a perpetual relaxation mode. (Granted, that was much better than perpetual violent waves of peristalsis.) Fortunately, it was not a permanent thing. It had just been a case of **aperistalsis**. You remove the little plug, finish the digital evacuation, and the rest was history. The digital evacuation seemed to stimulate the return of peristalsis.

Another intestinal phenomenon was, the little "pull" I would feel at the left side of the descending colon. Very unusual, when you consider I have no feeling in the rest of my abdomen. This was going to be another one of those annoying mysteries. (As a young nurse, I would secretly wonder about people who seemed to have nothing better to do, than count their bowel movements, after they retired. I had promised myself that I would not have that "hang-up." Of course, many had real problems; while, most just needed to correct their diets. As I became older and wiser, I realized that everything slows down, with age. Even the parts of a car, will wear out, with time.) Well, here we go: With the little "pull," would be this hardened lump right in the middle of my normal soft-formed stool. (Obviously, I had a "*hang-up*.") The little "pull" would feel like a burning rip, as it came loose. This might be a normal happening for some, but it was something new for me.... starting right after the incident. I'm thinking that perhaps the lining on a small spot in the colon had fused to the lining of the cavity. Perhaps, but with time the scar should heal and the membranous coating return. (Much as the spot burned on the nasal septum had healed.) It seemed, this spot was dry, and everything was having trouble, sliding pass. At first, it only occurred every few months; then, every couple of months; then, on to every month. (After nine years, a sigmoidoscopy was ordered to check the spot and no disease was found. So, it is just another little *mystery* I learn to live with. They were just more false messages, being sent by the brain.) I guess we need to be aware that, these things can happen anytime. It is simply another symptom we must watch for, in order to prevent obstructions or perforations. Of course, my doctors had a standard suggestion for both phenomena; try fiber therapy. ***There are more things to consider, in my case. All fiber therapies, warned against using their products, if you have any difficulty with swallowing. I have an allergy that causes my tongue and throat to swell. Perhaps, this is not the right therapy for me.*** Even though prunes are an irritant-laxative to me, I will use them; if necessary.

If that weren't enough, we still have this: Imagine the Water Resource People calling to say that they were sorry about the flood; the dam had broken. They will send a check. Too bad! I've had occasions, where the dam burst forth with a flood of water, and there was no stopping it. No checking this! There was no warning; no feeling of urgency; no bladder infection. The urethral sphincter was not doing the job… another false message from the brain. This has only happened a half dozen times over a six year period, but it is another problem that would tend to make you afraid of leaving your house, if you let it. You say to yourself, "How can I be sure this won't happen again?" But then, you say, "What makes you believe it ever will?!" You go on with your life. Let's face it, my friends and relatives will be as surprised to find out about these *little problems*, as you. Polite people don't speak of unmentionables. All of we Traumatic Brain Injury patients, need to be aware of these possibilities.

* * * * * * *

When I look back at my notes, I'm reminded of the many obstacles I experienced while trying to get on with my activities of daily living. Yet, maybe my weaknesses are what made me strong. There abides a real fighter somewhere inside this empty shell. I was determined that I would not let this get the better of me. Against unbelievable odds, I forged on.... even convincing my doctors that I should be allowed to return to work on a trial basis. Nursing was as natural as breathing, to me. I felt that I could work by osmosis. (Of course, I hadn't the ability to use logic. Logic would have told me to rest and regain some semblance of normalcy, before trying to return to work.) Working in a fog of slow motion, with delayed reactions and attention deficit was like a person on crutches, constantly having them kicked out from under them. Others cannot help you, if they don't understand the problems associated with SHOCK. You feel as though you are crossing this long, swaying footbridge; always unsure of your next step. For my good health, I probably should not have been working at all. But, it is natural; in life, we are constantly challenging ourselves to do better and climb higher. Perhaps, for the *Challenged*, it is not so important to climb higher as it is to simply climb.

Dare to dream! Though I kept asking when I was going to get back to my old self, any progress came slowly. At two and a half years, came obvious improvements that were all mine. I could claim them as something new. Maybe they won't seem like much to you, but I found the return of DREAMS and GOOSEBUMPS brought me back to *normal*... things that normal people do. Like a toddler who had just created his first miracle in the bathroom, I had passed another major hurtle on that road to life. And, I was so proud! I announced it to everyone. (Though, I don't know why; it's not from anything I did. The improvements, like the SHOCK, just happened.) I suppose this was part of the childish feelings I had from the decreased inhibitions. I see the reality now. What did I expect? It was not their problem. They are too involved in their own lives, to worry about mine. And, that is as it should be. As a couple of the doctors explained: My IQ remained, so why would anyone care about my lost abilities? "If the truth be told, many would even be happy about your predicament. Yes!! How many people sit around saying they would like to do something or go someplace special someday, but they never do it? They could be a little jealous of your accomplishments. (Why? When they reach my age, they will have accomplished a few more things, also.) No one cares if you can no longer fly an airplane or continue the underwater photography; never mind your inability to retain new information needed to continue your career. They were sorry the *electrocution* happened and will be more cautious about any electrical equipment; but that was in the past. At present, they don't care!" I needed to *Get a Grip*!

I'm expecting there will be more improvements over the coming years. I will welcome them, if and when they come; but I will not sit here and wait for them. I had not been able to dream or daydream for two and a half years; then, it happened. When I dreamed, it was in black and white. I used to dream in color. It's a start! I'll take what I can get. Of course, I couldn't remember what they were about, but I dreamed. (Years later, the dreams are rarities; they seldom visit. Perhaps the dreams are really there, but Short-Term-Memory robs me of their existence.) The goose bumps and the ability to feel "chilled" were unexpected, but somehow signaled a real improvement. Maybe this empty shell, without feeling a heart or soul, knows there is something inside, after all! I can feel nothing in this VOID. Yet,

I'M ALIVE, THEREFORE, I AM !

☺

CHAPTER 7

ONLY A

HEARTBEAT AWAY.

ONLY A HEARTBEAT AWAY.

One of the unwanted affects of my shock, was the pain we supposed to be Cardiac in nature. Since I had no sensation under my ribcage, how would we know? It may have been sub-sternal, but the pain was on top of the breastbone. We were pretty sure of the pain and pressure on the front of the throat, lower neck and left shoulder and arm. The EKGs were usually clipping along at 140-150; enough to give anyone angina. With this, I was so weak and tired, I became winded just walking across the room. At my young age and being in such great condition, I had never expected to be bothered by angina. I had been doing everything right; getting plenty of exercise and watching my diet. I don't use tobacco or alcohol. I don't understand! The pain was pretty intense. Sure, I would be sent to see the Hospitals' Insurance Company Doctors… no hurry… just, whenever they could fit me in; despite the racing heart rate and chest pain. Everything was in slow-motion and I hadn't had any experience with Workers Compensation before. What did I know? I thought it was normal procedure, to see the Company doctors, (though Workers Comp might have preferred I see doctors of their choosing). I thought that this was what I had to do, in order to receive treatment for my injuries, from Workers Comp. Still, I knew that I needed to see a Cardiologist on my own. I should not have waited two days, much less two months! At ten days, I phoned a specialist and was seen immediately.

The Cardiologist was amazed at my treatment, or lack thereof. I should have been kept in the hospital for observation and treatment of the Tachycardia. Cardiac Arrest will usually happen a day or two later; not necessarily at the time of the injury. He began my treatment with Cardiac drugs. If one didn't stop the problem, another one was tried, until we found the right one for me. I was taken off work, until seen by a Neurologist. (I wonder why the Hospital hadn't done that! SURE! They had insisted that I work or call in sick. And I was warned that I should not use too many sick days; after all, I was working "on-call." To be used when needed. And, it was the busy Holiday Season.) Still, I wonder how they could allow me to work in that condition. True, Nursing was like breathing to me, but the slow absorption of information and slow reaction time, can't be good. We won't even mention my health: (This obviously was not a priority for the Hospital), the tachycardia, probable angina, and shortness-of-breath, were pretty evident.

I made an appointment with a Neurologist, and went in for an evaluation. Of course, I didn't like what I heard. "Any improvement could take months, with optimal improvement taking years." I have always been an impatient person and have never liked "playing-a-waiting-game" with anything. I guess I knew, deep in my heart, that only time would tell the real story. In denial, I talked the Neurologist into letting me try working, "How can I know if my brain is working or not, if I don't use it?" You see, this doesn't decrease your IQ; just the ability to use it as effectively. I couldn't stand staying at home and looking at four walls all day. She agreed to let me work a trial day each week, to see how it went. (She probably thought that I would realize I was wrong, going back to work so soon.) We did need the money. No one can fully understand the determination I possessed. "What nobody else can do, I can." I would too, or die trying! I stubbornly persisted in dragging myself around in this unbelievable stupor, not understanding what was really happening; always thinking, "Maybe tomorrow, I'll be back to where I was before the SHOCK." Everything was in slow-motion. (I hadn't the sense to know any better.) The doctor had even cautioned me about not getting paid for the days lost from work or my medical bills, if I returned to work so soon. Hey, I'm a

Nurse. I know that old ploy. We've used it often enough. A patient has the right to refuse treatment, but they need to know that their insurance may not pay their bills, if they do refuse the doctors orders. This way, they can make an educated decision. This is a patient's right. (What can the facts do for someone with Attention Deficit and Short Term Memory? Could I decipher the information and make an appropriate decision? Not likely! After all, I am just ***Running on Neutral***, here.) But, SHE was right, of course. I really needed someone to hold me down and talk some sense into my head. Fat Chance! Not in this state of confusion. All I could think of is, we really needed the money now, and "on-call," I wouldn't get paid for sick days. In this FOG, I really wasn't making sense. I had it all wrong; in more ways than one. Little did I know, things would get a lot worse, before they got any better.

By now, I had seen the Company Doctors, who had done a good job and pretty much concurred with my Cardiologist and Neurologist. Though the 24 hour Cardiac Monitor was a waste. I was told to keep a diary of when I had pain and what my activity was. I did an accurate job. There was everything from pain in my throat and biceps, with nausea and weakness on that long drive home; to chest pain and shortness-of-breath during my walk. When I returned the Monitor, it was discovered that the time on the monitors clock was off twenty minutes. They would leave a note to that effect and adjust the time accordingly. There were all sorts of dysrhythmias, but nothing coincided with any of the problems in my diary. SURE! **I guess we know what happened there!**

Don't you know, a meeting was called by the Insurance Representative and my bosses. The Boss said that there was no reason, I couldn't return to full-time work. "Wait a minute," I protested. "Your doctors concurred with my doctors, and it was decided that I could try working, with certain restrictions." The Insurance Rep continued the bold-face-lie, "I have the full report right here, and there are no restrictions." I insisted that she show me the report. "It's right here," she said, as she flipped the paper back and forth under my nose. I knew what the doctors had said, so "Show me," I replied. There it was, in black and white; as I pointed to the note, I read it aloud. The meeting was over. I believe they thought they could take advantage of my condition. Too bad they didn't understand the Condition! (Is that paranoia?) "On-call" to be used as needed, or abused when possible? Besides, she had not yet received all of the Doctor's Reports! Yes, I resent the lack of *honor*; but then, this would not have been a word in her vocabulary. (As my brother would say, "Consider the source.") I may not remember everything that I hear, but I take notes and review the significant items. Strange, but some things are retained in my computer brain; just not available for selective recall.

I will have gone on having irregular heartbeats, slow heartbeats, fast heartbeats, and combinations of all of the above. In 1995, four years after the SHOCK, I would be in three ERs, in three different cities, to rule-out heart attacks. Each time, the Enzymes came back negative. I would go through Thallium Tests, Echocardiograms, and a Cardiac Cath. The small area of non-reperfusion in the apex, (which showed up on the Thallium Stress Test, given after my first episode of Chest Pain), was due to a narrowed left descending artery; BUT, only a 20% block, "which is nothing." Then why the pain? The diagnosis was determined to be "Syndrome X." I have been on the right medication for years, and there is no problem with chest pain, or *whatever*. I often wonder if I would feel it, if I really had chest pain. Probably not. I have no feeling, under the ribcage, at all! The pain on my back and on the right side of my chest, had to be treated as Cardiac, but my Cardiologist had just finished a battery of test, declaring me cardiac healthy. He sent me for an Ultrasound of the abdomen, for the *Atypical Chest Pain*. I had a very typical gallstone. The stone was removed, along with the gallbladder. And, with my continuing prophylactic medication for the Syndrome X, the pains were gone.

Inside this Empty Shell, there is a void. Though the current had traveled across my diaphragm, it kept functioning. I couldn't feel the rise and fall of my chest, but it was obviously happening; ....I was still alive. I just can't feel my lungs. Along with the numbness of the nostrils, back of the throat, and roof of the mouth, I have had some mighty big respiratory infections; both upper and lower. My dentist made me aware of one case of pneumonia. My throat was fire-red, but beyond that was the pneumonia. The other was found by my husbands insistence on my seeing the doctor. Another case of bronchitis and pneumonia! It's difficult, seeing a doctor when you have no pain. (However, I was becoming quite weak.) I soon learned, when I lose my voice, it's time to see the doctor. See, I'm finding new coping mechanisms! The bad part about not feeling the lungs is, you can't feel the congestion coming on. So, I've learned to listen for the barking cough, laryngitis, and the indisputable evidence being coughed up. Gross!

Another disruption to my daily routine came with my lifelong allergy to smoke. I had learned avoidance, or seeking fresh air when coming into contact with smoke. That had always worked well for me. Back in the days when some nurses smoked, I can't have been too popular, when they would have to snuff-out their cigarettes during report, at the change-of-shift. (I don't know why I was embarrassed and apologized for their inconvenience. If we keep up this rate of pollution, we will all be wearing SCABA instead of SCUBA. That is self-contained above-water breathing apparatuses.) This sensitivity became much worse, after the Near-Electrocution. I had to have an inhaler and antihistamine; and an EPI-pen for emergencies. I could not stay around those who smelled of strong cigarette smoke. It got to the point, I would have to have someone watch my patients for me, while I took my medication and got my breathing back to normal. Granted, it was a rare occasion. There were a few other nurses with asthma, so we thought nothing of covering for one another.

Our home was in a Pleasant Town valley. Coming home at midnight, we would sink into smoke so thick, you could cut it with a knife. What a miserable night that would bring! The Pleasant Town finally cleaned-up-it's-act, after we moved over the hill to a smaller, cleaner town. Guess what! A few years "over the hill" and we found ourselves in a *Boom*; one of the fastest growing cities in California. Now, our New Town is thick with smoke. We can always hope that New Town will ban wood-burning fireplaces, also.

Before my Near-electrocution, I could always tell when I needed to get to clean air, as my tongue and throat would start to swell. At present, I can be so bad, my neck looks like it has a noose around it, before I realize I need medication. The throat is numb. I feel nothing, but I can see my tongue. There have been some scary incidents! We do take our good health for granted. I never had trouble detecting the problem before. Just like the pneumonia, we have to listen for symptoms: me to start clearing my throat; or, I know whenever I have difficulty swallowing .... a much advanced symptom ....it's time to act. Worse yet, is when we have a Bad Air Day (usually due to the ozone) and I wake up at night, with the enlarged tongue, swelling around the neck, and difficulty getting my breath, or swallowing the pills. Sure, I tease about all of the "Cabin Fever," but know that I have to stay inside during the Bad Air Days and during the cool weather, when the neighbors throw a log on their fireplaces (though, the particles from wood-burning fireplaces are small enough to go through your walls). Only someone with Asthma or other breathing problems, can appreciate this struggle. These statistics are growing, at an alarming rate.

I guess I would be in denial, if I said I wasn't concerned about not feeling my insides. Of course, I think there could be things going wrong and I would not catch the symptoms in time to do anything about it, but you push that onto the back burner. As a positive person, I would like to ignore negativity. You know how I hate playing waiting games, yet, I do have to second-guess every dry cough or croup. Was that spot they found on my x-ray significant or just a poor picture? I must say, I really don't want any more x-rays; I'm already glowing in the dark. So it will remain just another *sweet mystery of life.* You could let your imagination go wild, but what would that accomplish? Still, you must be vigilant, with prudent preventive care. (I wonder if A *TOTAL BODY SCAN* might be appropriate, every 5-10 years, for someone with these injuries.) It would be nice to know, that no new problems have occurred. Then again, we do have to allow for my allergies to diagnostic DYES!

Even my allergies to medications and food have become more prevalent and more difficult to detect. We can pretty well guess that if my abdomen suddenly bloats like a nine-month pregnant woman, I probably have enteritis, "Stop the allergy medication." Nausea and vomiting is easily detected; the fast, irregular, and thready pulse, is only detected, when I feel weak. "STOP" that antibiotic or suppository. While it may be true, that Blondes have more fun; they usually have more allergies, also. Suddenly, I've become sensitive to almost everything; even certain foods, I'd never had trouble with before the SHOCK. (There is a strange reversal here: the antibiotics and foods my youngest son is allergic to, I have now become allergic to.) I will need to approach any new item with caution. I guess my husband has had enough surprises, with my reactions to new medications. We have a deal: I will never start another medication, unless he is there to observe the outcome. We start it on a weekend, so he can observe me for a day or so. My husband has learned the hard way. You may say he is overly protective, but his caution has proved life-saving, time and again. He and I are both more comfortable, since he took the CPR course. A history of allergic reactions, along with that lifelong allergy to smoke, has taught us caution. The great outdoors is my preference, anyway. (Just watch out for forest fires.) You see, precaution and avoidance had become a way of life, much like every Asthma Patient. I can handle this. I just need to know what to look for, if that's possible.

I've had two instances of classic "Cushings Syndrome." The only explanation from all three doctors was "An allergic reaction to something." No one could guess WHAT. I found that wild! Who would think that an allergic reaction would cause swelling of the trunk, only? Weird things happen. No one knows better than I. This whole experience has been an on-going revelation.

I am now sensitive to barley. Not too unusual, but do you realize that they are putting barley flour in everything, from bread to cereals?! Then, there is my old allergy to Nutra-sweet. If you think airline food is bad, just try reading the list of ingredients on those little wrappers. I don't care if it is a cookie or a sandwich, I must read the labels. (My husband shares P.I. Duty.) I like the sugar-free gum with a list of ingredients a mile long; starting with dextrose, and ending with aspartame. Sure, my ears were killing me, but it was not a favor you did for me, when you offered the piece of gum that, "doesn't contain Nutra-Sweet." It would have been better to have had painful ears, than to stagger off of the plane. It occurred to me, many do not understand that **Nutra-Sweet** and **aspartame** are one and the same. Don't be taken- in by every new miracle product that comes along. Of course, they are going to say that there are no side-effects, (they're liars, and) they are just trying to sell their products. The fact remains that anything you put in your mouth or eyes, on your skin, or suppository, etc. is still a foreign object and can cause reactions! So, don't fall for their ads so completely, that you overlook the possibility of reactions.

The same is true of Splenda; check their claims! Anything different, can cause a problem.

Another big-time allergy: YELLOW DYES give me Tachycardia; a heart rate like the feet of a racing horse. Again, found in everything from cereal to Tylenol Gelcaps. (And, can the makers of Dyazide tell me why a white capsule needs yellow dye?) Thirty percent of the population is sensitive to yellow dyes; and, I'm told, another thirty percent are sensitive to red dyes. Let's see, what color would enteric coatings be? Red? Orange? Yellow? Or, all of the above? Which leads me to wonder if sensitivities to the medications, are due to the medicine or it's coloring. Who would ever know?

I, like most adults, am on a low-dose aspirin each day, for cardiac health. Since I cannot use enteric coated ones or orange-flavored ones, because of their yellow dyes, I use the cherry-flavored chewables. If any of your family members are sensitive to dyes, you may want to check out the cheese puffs and taco chips you buy the family. We need healthier, not prettier foods. Pay attention, PUBLIC. When we start paying attention, the food and pharmaceutical processors will pay attention. Don't look for the dye contents on the bottles. They are on the box, the bottle came in. You know, the one you threw in the trash. You would think that the ingredients would be printed on the bottles; but then, have you ever tried to read the dosage instructions? No room for more words.

Now, I am allergic to **benzalkonium chloride**. This is a simple antiseptic used in most nasal sprays. So much for my sinus problems! The decongestant sprays prescribed, contain benzalkonium chloride, while the pills and capsules contain yellow dyes. Sometimes, you just can't win. I'd be in real trouble, without saline. Most eye drops, also contain benzalkonium chloride. How about eye exams? Today, we have Optomap. A laser picture is taken of the entire eye, decreasing the need to dilate, those allergic to the drops.

New foods and drugs which can cause problems, are many. Again, I will have to approach any new item with caution. However, some doctors didn't seem to get the message; the various ulcer and reflux medications were ineffective. But then, these medications often work with your gastric parietal lining to be effective, and **mine had been fried**. One can see how allergies and sensitivities could increase tremendously. I am not of the same make-up, as before. This infused heat has altered my whole being. However, nutrients are being absorbed, so healing is taking place.

This book is not long enough to list every allergy, but just a sample might be: skin lotions, soaps, make-up, sun blocks, talc, *Plus* ingredients in antibiotic ointments, *New, Improved* toothpaste or laundry detergent, *Added benefits* for smoother skin (like PABA, Titanium Dioxide, cocoa butter, and Retin-A). I am always skeptical, when someone has *New and Improved* Products; you can bet they have just ruined a good thing. The toothpaste, laundry detergent, and skin lotion I'd been using for years, have dropped by the wayside, after the *New/Improved* versions came out. Is nothing sacred? We may as well talk about the new round handles on the toothbrushes. Just wrap your carpal tunnel hand around one of those babies! Ouch! My dentist can't use rubber gloves; my gums break-out. Nylon clothing is one of those "Don't even think about it!" subjects. Shrimp and seafood are forbidden. With most fresh fruits and vegetables, along with tomato sauce and <u>chocolate</u>, *I'm home free*; so, life is pretty good, after all.

Hey, but, science moves on! There is always something new coming down the pike. Many researchers are working on reasons why some people seem to be more susceptible to allergies than others. There may be a shot one day, that can limit our body's response to allergens. Wouldn't that be nice?

Understanding our DNA can solve many mysteries. (It would only be a matter of time.) We've all read about these on-going *Medical Miracles*. With pharmacogenomics, a whole new world is opening up to us. They can now, do a test on your DNA for TPMT, an enzyme that helps break down certain drugs. More than 100,000 Americans die each year, from adverse reactions to medications. Mutations of specific genes can interfere with your body's ability to metabolize these drugs; or, may even accelerate metabolism. We <u>will</u> have personalized medicine. We need only to be genotyped. Soon, your doctor will be able to adjust the proper dosage of each medication, specifically for you. He may be able to raise your dosage, lower your dosage, or avoid the drug, all together. This is truly a genomic revolution. I hope it is as good as it sounds. With all of the adverse reactions I've had to medications, it would be good to know ahead of time, what my genes are doing. This could save a lot of guess-work for everyone; and, guarantee a good nights' sleep for my husband and family. Check on the specifics of the TPMT test, on the web. You can check May 2004 Reader's Digest, also.

* * * * * * *

When it comes to most sensitivities, I think we will find

Pollution Connections. Years ago, we could just ignore the poisoning of our lakes and streams, thinking out-of-sight meant the problem was gone; only to have it raise it's ugly head, years later, in the food we eat. (Mercury Poisoning)

We have poured, and continue to pour tons of pollution into the air we breathe. (Childhood Asthma is at an all-time high.)

Polluted Air is also associated with cardiac problems! (Though, I guess that makes sense; if it is harder to breathe, that would cause increased work on your heart.) Like the *canary in the mine*, when will we ever learn, if not now? We must open our minds, before we can open our eyes to see.

* * * * * * *

Here is a poem, that was given to me.

SO WHAT ?!!!

Mama, what has happened with this *Silent Spring*?
Have you noticed, there are no birds to sing?
I don't know what has happened to most forms of life,
but, this silence cuts just like a knife.

I'm hungry, Mama; what can we eat?
The fields were scorched by the Summers heat.
Our Synthetic food is getting low.
I don't know how much further it will go.

Why did my brother have to die?
There is no ozone in the sky.
Authorities warned us to stay inside,
but little boys don't know to hide,
from a sun that can cook them, as they play.
That's what took your brother away.

***Remember to put on your solar gear,
before you go out to play;
and the re-breather pack upon your back,
will keep you safe, that way.***

I know mama. The temperature can melt gold,
but we look just like those "*bugs-of-old.*"
In my books, I can see,
Bugs that look just like we.

Where did my Daddy go?
He was caught in the twelve-foot snow.
It flash-froze everything exposed.
Even though, it was only June,
still, the snow, it came too soon.

When the snow melted, the hills turned to clay.
That is why we feel earthquakes, from miles away.
Is that why our cities have disappeared?
I'm afraid it is much more than that, my dear.

Our Great Lakes are greater than we could envision.
Elevated waters, are just one of the reasons.
Our continent is divided, by this vast waterway.
(Called *The Mighty Mississippi*, back in our day.)

The Gateway Arch is an *obstacle to navigation*.
What has become of this once-great nation?
While no one could harness nature, that's true;
but, wasn't there anything man could do?

Miami is gone (with the rest of the State).
New Orleans, a memory of similar fate.
New York City? That was one gigantic quake!!
The Continental Shelf couldn't take the weight.

Texas is disappearing, at an alarming rate.
Why, you wouldn't even recognize it, by its' shape.
California tumbled into the sea.
(This was predictably.)
Their mountains have become their only escape.

The deserts are oceans of water and sand.
Even the Grand Canyon has filled up again!
We could count on Rain Forest, for life-giving rain;
Clean water to drink, but do they remain?
We've destroyed them all, to our real shame.

The satellites verify, no snowcaps remain;
water covers, an indisputably, larger domain.
Only mountains and hills protrude from the depths.
We've become a people so inept;
there was *no winning;*
having returned our sphere to liquids and gases,
as In The Beginning.

Hurricanes are massive; tornadoes abound;
volcanoes are erupting, all around.
Earthquakes and Hail Storms, from every direction;
like, these vengeful floods,
have caused intolerable afflictions.

We tried drinking water, made from our oceans.
But, the rotting flesh soon canceled that notion.
Our skin is full of boils, from contact, of course.
We can't even bathe, in this foul-smelling source.

Europe is cold and Chili is hot!
I don't understand this mysterious plot.
None can survive, in either place.
Just, what has happened to our Earth's Face?

I'm haunted by the words of prophecy:
They were so blind, they would not see.
Stubbornly claiming their fantasy,
of Natural" changes, that will be.

Mama, It seems the whole Earth is being
RE-FORMED.
It's a shame the people hadn't been.
The warnings were there.
We might have saved this civilization,
if someone had cared.
Shall we run out and play,
while we still have another day?

We must always remember our solar shields
and re-breather packs.

Who would have guessed, it would come to that?
No house could withstand these storms, so great.
So, we'll sit in our caves and helplessly
wait.....................

SOOOOOOOoo WHAT!!!

by permission
WELCH WYNN-WHITE
Nov. 1, 1999

AHEAD OF THE GAME.

Like the heart, my neurological problems got worse, the first few weeks. I would like to talk about the head, rather than the end results. As a nurse, I could understand the false messages being sent by the brain (the Hives and Welts, etc.), but I had real difficulty with the strange phenomena I would encounter with the skull. I suppose, it would be expected that the burning would get worse. It felt as if my brain was being soaked in very warm bathwater. There was unbelievable pressure on the back of the head. (It actually felt like someone was pushing on the back of my head with their hand.) Then, it felt like my head was swollen like a big pumpkin.

The pain in the top of the head was burning hot and deep. There were definite spots of pain, about an inch deep, at the margins of the parietal and the frontal areas. One on the right and one on the left. It seemed as though Rolando's Fissure was fused. Confusing? If a worker flexed their flux and dropped a glob of solder right in the middle of a major circuit board, it would be ruined. They would have to replace it. I can't replace mine. I'm stuck with the damaged circuitry. (Perhaps, if I don't put too much demand on the functioning parts, I won't blow a fuse.) The right side seemed more severe a burn than the left. When we consider the injuries to the Occipital, Parietal, and Frontal Lobes, one wonders how I survived. (As I look over the pictures in my Logs, I'm amazed.) Of course, my first reaction to the burning in my Occipital Area was, "Thankfulness for my sight." Those first few days, when the burning became worse, I wondered if my sight would suffer. Would the pressure build-up cause a problem? Sometimes the pressure was so great, it felt like my head would pop. I look at the pictures and realize how close the burns came to the midbrain; everything seemed to miss the vital areas. THANK GOD!

The burns in the top of the head, were the most bothersome. There were episodes of jabbing pain from out of nowhere. It felt like someone had pushed an ice pick through the top of my head. Sometimes, it would shoot along the top of the frontal lobe to above the eyebrow. When the radiating pain persisted, there would be a headache and photophobia. The pain would be so great, it would cause the eye to squint. With the increased TOH (**T**op **o**f **H**ead Pain), came numbness of the cheeks, usually around the outside corners of the eyes. With the increased pain, came increased confusion. It was more difficult to think. (I had seen this with my Migraine Patients, also.) This was to be expected. But, the really bizarre phenomena came as the hives, "sunburn," or the red ears had appeared. We really couldn't understand these happenings. The lumps and bumps are a real curiosity. How does the brain do that?! My head is playing a "Head Game!" Again, no rhyme or reason; so it seemed to me. There was the bruise-like lump along the crest of the right side of the head… Occipital to Parietal to Frontal. It was a raised lump you could see and feel, but no discoloration. The bruise-like feeling was inside. There would be other "goose eggs." It seems they would build to a crescendo, over a week or two, then lightened. (What, an aseptic abscess? A pseudocyst? I don't know. Probably my *BRAIN* is playing another *im*practical joke.) Sometimes the "goose egg" would just be a big lump, right on the top of the head. With the increased swelling would come increased confusion, photophobia, facial numbness, and headaches.

We all like "baseball," don't we? Not the ball that would appear behind my right ear… like a three inch boil; we could see the lump, but no discoloration. Try sleeping, with a baseball tied to your head! Not an easy task. When these things got to the point you thought your head would explode, they would suddenly lighten. (Whatever the problem, we are not going in, to look for solutions. That would be all you needed, having an affinity for blood clots.) Every time you think you have this game-plan figured out, the rules change. One time, I had a "baseball" at the crown, right side superior parietal lobe. There were the usual symptoms of facial numbness, but let's add the right temporal area and orbital area. (I know, first hand, what a "numb skull" is.) The Occipital Pressure was unbelievable. As the pressure built, I became too hot; then, too cold; then, too hot again. This went on all night. Morning brought relief. Even though the right-sided pressure and pain were much worse than the left, usually; occasionally, the left side would become much stronger. Another change of the game-plan! (As expected.)

Yes, I still have the TOH and the OP (Occipital Pressure). Mostly right-sided. All symptoms are worse when I have a cold or am on antibiotics. As a matter of fact, I am having a big problem with the TOH and O/P right now; just, from being rundown. If I have lunch and come back to proofread where I left off, (because I won't remember), I will find sentences which are just another part of that big jig-saw puzzle. .... because I had no. We couldn't even ...the outcome. no.... WHAT? Even.... WHAT? The sentences were lost. I couldn't remember what the subject was, so they were deleted. (Have I expressed the difficulty involved, in writing this book?)

This was one of those days when I should have put off writing, for another time. Had I tried Solitaire first, I would have known that the ability to think, was not as sharp. I don't know if I will ever be *ahead of the game*, but I will work with it. I've accepted the fact that some things will never change. To some degree or another, the TOH with the cheek numbness, and the OP are always present. It has become a part of me. The Red Ears still light up like neon signs, when they appear. (What can I say? I have unusual talents.) Across my back, comes the Retro-Peritoneal

Burning to steal my sleep like a nasty sunburn; though it is a rare occasion, now. The "goose eggs" will visit, now and then. For me, there is no keeping ahead of the game. But, I'll take the cards I'm dealt. I will not "Fold." I'm playing my hand to the end of the game!! So, don't count me out. Like the other *sweet mysteries* in my life, I hope to laugh at these novelties one day; but, I find nothing funny about them, while they are in progress.

* * * * * * *

Should I even attempt making sense of any of this? I don't think I can. *Houston* might say, "All systems GO," while I'm tempted to say, "All systems are GONE." Though all systems were affected, none of the organs were completely dysfunctional. (Though, some are real Rouges!) The Current had moved over the diaphragm; still, it functioned: I'm breathing! The brain is still taking care of my autonomic needs, in it's own way. When something like this happens, you are made aware, once again, that death is *Only A Heartbeat Away*; while you are striving to stay *Ahead Of The Game,* you are vulnerable to that *Split Second.*

* * * * * * *

CHAPTER 8

COPING MECHANISMS

COPING MECHANISMS...

How does one cope with life's problems? We all have our own little idiosyncrasies: Our own special ways of coping. We have gathered them throughout our lifetime. We have amassed a store of mechanisms, ready to cope with anything thrown our way; surely, they will always be there. Not necessarily! It's another realm we take for granted. One doesn't miss them until they are gone. Think of everything you would be giving up, if you were to lose your coping mechanisms. Erase them all! Your ability to function in the *Real Adult World* is hampered, because you are like a child learning to cope all over again. Think about it. This will have an effect on all facets of your life. Having my very essence ripped away, coping became impossible; and, **"Just when I needed it most!!!"** With my added challenges of Attention Deficit and Short-Term Memory Retention, I am left with this void! Once again, A void is nothing, but it goes on forever.

Are you the type who finds solace in reading? Well, I cannot read self-help books, calming poetry, magazines, news of the world, or anything else, for that matter. So, on top of feeling empty inside, I feel isolated in my condition. At first, I couldn't even finish reading a complete sentence; I will have forgotten the first part of the sentence, by the time I would reach the end of the sentence. (And I was used to reading three newspapers a day.) Well-meaning friends and acquaintances would hear me tell them I could not read or retain information; then, they would inform me of helpful books I should read! (Yes, I know, "Many will listen, but few will hear.") I have improved somewhat, over the years. I can read short articles and usually remember them, for the day. Hearing a cute joke on TV, I will have to write it down quickly, if I want to share it with someone else. I do retain things I hear better than things I read; though, not for long. If this had happened years ago, I would have been a cheap date. One could buy a good video, make some popcorn, and we could see the same mystery over and over... it would still be a thriller to me. We have a joke in this family: you don't send her to the video store to rent a movie. She will get the one we saw last week! (Now, the video store will check their computer, for our previous rentals. This way, I don't rent the same ones twice.) I still find it difficult admitting to anyone, that I have this problem of short-term memory.

Recently, I received a card, informing me of an over-due movie. I called the store and told them we had not rented that movie. He pulled up our record on the computer and told me exactly when and what two movies we had rented. The one sounded familiar, but the second title was unfamiliar. I asked if it was one that we had to return as defective. If not, what was it about? I don't remember that! He goes into more detail. (Of course, none of this is familiar to me.) I do remember something about the defective one he took back; it had so many four-letter words anyway, that you would need an interpreter. The poor guy was reciting the story-line of every movie. I finally told him that he was talking to the woman with brain injury and short-term memory. "But it seems to me, if my husband returned the one movie, he would have returned the other one at the same time. One was checked in at 10:00 AM and the other after the noon deadline; at which time he would be eating his lunch, getting ready for work. I would guess that the store was behind at checking in the returns." Suddenly the guy who was trying to get a thief to pay for a stolen movie, quietly said that everything was alright. I should tell my husband that everything was okay. (I guess he figures, my husband has enough problems!) Why can't I admit my disability? Worse yet, why do I get myself into these situations? That darn 20-Minute Delay! I received the card in the mail on the sixteenth and it requested that we reply on or before the sixteenth. My husband was at work, so I replied. Duh! Is the world going to come to an end, if we respond on the seventeenth? I thought I would do my husband a favor. When will I learn that I get into trouble, being so helpful? And, I don't know why I bother recording TV movies, we've already seen nine-tenths of them. We may have a treasure-trove of VHS movies, but who would know, since I forget to write the name of the movie on the label? Still, *Hope Springs Eternal.* (Every experience happens for a reason. We learn the lesson being taught, by acting to accept or reject a premise. Though, for the past nine years, I had worked at hiding my disabilities, this was the day I determined to talk freely about my specific "challenges." They will not be disabling, but rather, set me free.)

I was always the type who thirsted for knowledge. My parents taught us that ***we need not know a lot about anything,* but *we should know a little bit about everything.*** The thirst filled my life. I could be driving along and hear something on the radio that didn't seem right, (Did I say I was born in Missouri?) so, it was not unusual for me to pull into the library and research the subject. Sometimes, I was right. Other times, I learned something new. How I wish I still possessed that ability. (Couldn't I have given this Workers Comp Hell?!!! As I think about it now, I'm sure there must have been some infringement of my Civil Rights and the Disability Act. Lucky for them, I can't fight!) I'm unable to concentrate, attention is short with disorganized thought processes, and I have short-term memory retention. Researching anything is a wash-out. This had been another coping mechanism. Everyone loves to read. Reading gives you a connection with the rest of the world. I used to keep up with *the latest*, but now, the world is passing me by. I'm really feeling separated from everyone else, until I consider the many adults who cannot read. I know how they must feel. For non-readers it's a scary and lonely place. Strange, isn't it? I always wanted to teach adults to read, when I retired. All I can do now, is encourage others to do so.

In my depths of despair, we lost the family dog. In a shocking surprise, we returned from vacation to pick up our dog from the kennel, only to find him in convulsions, dying. A shock on top of my SHOCK. We could say, "Adding insult to injury." This dog was supposed to have a longevity of twenty years. He was five years old! You say, "Surprise?" Why surprise? Because, twice we had called and checked on him, long distance. He was doing fine, eating well, playing ball, and taking his walks. Our plane arrived too late for us to pick him up on Friday night, so we called to check on him again and to tell them we would pick him up in the morning, as previously planned. Again, he was "fine." This dog was our connection with the family we had left behind in another state. Something we had in common. He was like another child. I could laugh with him, play with him, tease him, and scold him. Through it all, you knew when you came home after a hard night's work, Ralff was there to listen or just sit quietly by. He had such a *calming effect* on us. Another useful coping mechanism.

I couldn't understand why I was taking his death so badly. I found myself crying over this dumb animal! Maybe that was the problem... he wasn't a dumb animal. I felt there was some sort of connection. Just as my husband said, "He seemed to sense what we were thinking." At any rate, my husband soon put his finger on the problem. I had not been able to mourn his absence or his missed qualities.

I was the poet of the family; an anniversary, birthday, eulogy, or special occasion; they could count on me. As a song writer, my brother *just had the music* in his head. I've always thought in rhyme. I didn't know that this was unusual. I believed everyone thought in rhyme. I couldn't understand why some students were so apprehensive about writing poems for English Class… "Just write down whatever comes to you." Anyway, the poetry had been another unknown coping mechanism in my life. Now, I know what I'm missing. I had not been able to write about the dogs passing; and when my husband pointed out this fact, I understood that my grieving was normal.

The loss of the family pet had been so painful, we lasted about six weeks before getting another puppy. He was no Ralff, but he had talents of his own; and breaking-in a new dog kept us occupied. This Pup could bound five feet straight up in the air, from a standing position. I have never seen a dog do that. However, when we bathed him, beneath all of that long fluffy hair, were the muscles of a Pit Bull. When we moved into the new house (with it's lovely light-beige carpeting), he bounded up onto the kitchen counter and found a package of chocolate cupcakes. You know how difficult they are to open! He had to struggle all over the living room, before getting them open. Then, he had to eat them out of those little plastic packing cups. When we returned home from a hard nights work, I cried. We were too tired for this, but we had no choice! It's not as if you could call a carpet cleaner at two o'clock in the morning. Knowing chocolate is poison for dogs, I called the Vet. "If he was alright now, he would probably be okay." This dog has become very considerate, once we trained him. Why, just today, he emptied the trash for me. Something Ralff never did. (However, Ralff did rearrange the flower beds quite often.) Once we had child-proofed the drawers and cabinets, gave him obedience lessons, established the "Time-Out" Room, and tied all of the laces together on each pair of our shoes (he can't inspect the inside of the shoes, if you keep them closed); we pretty well had <u>him</u> trained. As I look at this, I wonder ...why do we keep buying white dogs?! A pause for thought. My poetry had been such a great coping mechanism. Perhaps, just writing raw feelings down on a piece of paper, puts things in perspective. It really helps you see things more clearly. In poetic phrases, things seem less harsh. Reality less stinging.

Along with the loss of the poetic abilities, I became unable to use that old MIND-OVER-MATTER ploy. You know, the head doesn't really hurt, you just need to take a minute and relax; or, the blood pressure is up, well just let me chill-out a minute and take it again. If I had difficulty getting to sleep, I used self-hypnosis; you know, you start by telling your toes "Relax toes," "Relax feet," and work your way up. Somewhere along the way, you fall asleep. Not now; thoughts scatter. I no longer have that talent for deep concentration.

Perhaps my acquaintances didn't miss it, but I missed another weird ability I had possessed... extrasensory perception. Though I hadn't realized I was doing it, I would answer questions, before they were asked. I knew when the telephone was going to ring, AND who it was, And often what they wanted. The same was true for company coming. Not to mention, grabbing thoughts out of the air. That could be embarrassing! My friends will be glad to know, I am now normal, that way. Though they had marveled at the ESP, I'm slow to grasp the meaning of anything they say, today. Worse yet, I may not remember any of it, tomorrow. Another difficult thing for people to understand was, not remembering names. I can tell you the names of those I worked with before the incident; however, I will not remember the names of those I met after the incident. No offense. I found most of them amiable. How do I handle prayer? Not too well... the attention deficit is lousy. I've compensated by praying "Whenever." The one thing I could always count on, was the fact that God loves me and will always be there for me. I've found, no matter what befalls us, HIS grace is sufficient. Sure, I'm ashamed of my whining over this. Ours is not to reason why, but to see the good that can come from misfortune. Will it use you, or will you use it?

With decreased inhibitions, my problems were using me! Some of the newer coping mechanisms were **not me!** I cannot tell you how embarrassing this was! It was that delayed response/reaction time that caught me off-guard.

My so-called "**20 Minute Delay.**" As I was entering the expressway one day, the driver of a little pick-up truck decided this was his entrance at the last minute, and expected me to go over the embankment to let him into my lane. I had no place to go, so he had to slow and fall in behind me. As some insecure men have been known to rationalize their behavior by diverting the blame to others, he was no exception. Macho Madness! How dare I, not risk my life for him! I usually ignore these characters, but... he kept trying to run me off of the expressway, I remained in my lane; he would pull in front of me and brake, I would go around him in the other lane; he would speed up and get in front of me and brake again. His little wife was scared to death. This nut was going to cause an accident! This called for desperate measures! This peace-loving little lady, flipped him a bird like a pro. He took out like a bat. I guess he figured, if that crusty old broad was flipping birds, she could be crazy. It was embarrassing, but it worked. Talk about *learned behavior*... I used it again during another instance: a delivery truck pulled out of a driveway without looking. He honked and yelled at me. A bird was flying! End of the situation. However, I always felt guilty afterwards. Maybe that was just a deacon from the church, honking "Hello." No, I hadn't recognized the face. Or, the language. (Though, I should.) If my inhibitions were down, why didn't that include guilt? "Miss Prim and Proper" was using foul language. Where did that come from? I was not used to behaving so poorly; nor using slang. Being raised to believe only ignorant people resort to slang and harsh "shock" words to make a complete sentence. This was soooo beneath me! Sure. Now convince that driver!

I also found myself arguing like a ten-year-old. From my pre-teens, I had never seen a purpose for arguing. You state your position. They state their position. I let you be you. You let me be me. No need to argue. A matter of simple courtesy. I couldn't believe I was actually feeling things, I had not felt since childhood. If someone slandered me, I felt badly. Normally, an adult would just let something like that roll off their back, like water off a duck. I became confrontational. Once again, remembering my mothers teachings: "If a gossip is talking about you, they are giving someone else a rest." I do believe that, but still the feelings came. Maybe that is a part of the delayed response. You know, if you add the "Ifs," "Ands," and "Buts" to the equation, it would not bother you. Everyone has problems. Don't let their problems become yours. You never know the full story. Perhaps, they are the youngest or only child, raised as a "Princess," uncertain of their abilities or their gender, insecure in their job or love life, having money problems, needing attention, or having family distractions. The list goes on. My brother had a great way of summing things up, "Always consider the source!" Thankfully, I no longer "flip birds," or cuss so much; the wrong words still slip out, but at least I recognize them. That bent for arguing has passed. Coping might not have been such a job, had I been able to rid myself of those useless *delicate, hurt feelings.* What a waste of time. Being unable to control my feelings, floored me. I couldn't understand why anyone would bother with such junk. My poor brain needed to recapture more important things. The one useless feeling that remained, was the paranoia. That could take a while. I have been *taken-advantage-of* so many times during this incident, naivety has left me. Still, there is a reason for all things. Even at my age, I needed to know that, "Not everyone strives to live honorably." Once again, that is their problem, not yours. Remaining the cock-eyed optimist, I choose to see the best in people.

The wrong words may continue to plague me. If you and I were sharing the waiting room at the dentist, you probably wouldn't notice a problem. I can carry on a normal conversation. Who cares if the wrong words flow? You don't know me. I will not be accountable for remembering our conversation tomorrow. (Hopefully, you will not be there the next time I come in.... I won't remember you, much less our conversation!) While an occasional "damn" or "hell" will slip out, some would see this as normal. I enjoy getting out in public. Your conversation was enlightening, for the day. It gave me a lift. I may take home that great recipe you gave me, put it in my recipe box and, next week, "I wonder where the hell that came from." My family and friends find it amusing. I can't help it, but I don't have to like it.

For some reason, windmills became "Lawnmowers," and on occasion, "Wheelbarrows." **Where does that come from?!!!** If I were my old analytical self, I would be reasoning: Is the connection the turning wheels and blades, compound words, or the fact that they have so many of the same letters? I don't know! The real reason is probably the *SAME OLD, SAME OLD...*The brain is sending messages over a faulty pathway. There are rouges traveling my expressways, making a mockery of order. Some travel so fast, they haven't the ability to comprehend the dangers ahead. (Like my blurting-out, whatever comes to mind, without thinking. Some woman was loudly proclaiming the Lord's name. I spun around and shouted, "Where?" Like, it's any of my business! <u>Extremely</u> embarrassing! **What would I think** of these actions? Crazy! I'm putting forth an effort to re-socialize myself, but I'm not always in control.)

Many messages will wind up in a tangled wreck (without bringing any message at all), while others will make the detour around the maze of mangled nerves; moving along, but taking an alternate route with differing outcomes. (Like doing something before the 20-Minute Delay kicks in.) Either way, there are few to pick up the pieces. There are no cell phones calling for help; no emergency vehicle can reach the destination; no doctor can understand; no tests or drugs can help; and no amount of coping will change the outcome.

Someday, you hope to capture the rogues and put them away. In the least, hoping those on detour will arrive at the proper destinations with the appropriate message. We can only hope. (I started to say, "We can dream," but that is not an option; rather, a rarity.) I've learned to keep quiet and let the other person say the name of the subject: i.e., "Just look at this amazing beauty." Let them expound on the white windmills against the blue sky on the green rolling hills. Those who are familiar with my condition, understand and are able to laugh with me.

Still, the wrong words in a given situation, can be most embarrassing. Like the time a mother brought in her two-year-old son for an asthma treatment. As an ER Nurse, I would have to use ingenuity to get a child to wear those oxygen mask. In the days of the "Ninja Turtles," I could talk a child into using his mask by calling it a Ninja Turtle Mask. This child was too young to care. I told his mother not to be concerned. "We would just do a blow job." I had meant to say, "Blow-by;" a term we use for holding the child on your lap, while directing the oxygen toward their face. "Oops, the wrong words came out," I explained, with the red face. We all had a good laugh. Though I doubt it, the mother may forget what I said tomorrow, but strangely enough, something so embarrassing, "Miss Prim and Proper" is going to remember. That GUILT thing again! It could have been worse. It might have been the father with his son, or a male Respiratory Therapist present. The child might have been old enough to ask questions. I have to see the positive in all things.

See, you won't forget the embarrassing instances: One of the nurses was at lunch, so I checked-in one of her patients for her. The girl was there because her doctor said she had a bad case of *stomatitis* and needed to have it checked-out. I asked her how long she had had stomach problems. (I would guess that I had known for about forty years, that stomatitis has nothing to do with the stomach; it is an inflammation of the mouth.) Here I was again, with another computer glitch. With the delay in assimilation, I wouldn't notice the difference, for an hour or two. When it came to me, I had said such a ridiculous thing, I was embarrassed and humiliated. Talk about denial! We still feel ashamed, even if we are not in control of the Rogue Roads. I wonder if I'll ever get over that problem, completely. I look so normal, even I want to forget I'm not. It's a slow process, but when I can talk about my deficiencies, the embarrassment disappears; like a weight, being lifted off my shoulders. It is not my favorite subject, but there are times I need to *speak-up*.

"Well, my words escape me." No, really; my words do escape me! This happens with words I had used for years; even those that were an integral part of my life or job. I was asked by a psychologist to name the smallest blood vessels. (I can tell you, the first thing a Nurse does when she enters a patients room, is to check their color and capillary refill. Yet, here I was with another dropped computer chip.) I could name vessels, large and small; from the Vena Cava to the Aorta, and from the venules to arterioles, but it was as if the information about capillaries had been dropped completely. I had never heard of these strange things, of which he spoke. I didn't even recognize it *as a word!* When he explained it to me, I believed it existed. (Just, not in my mind!) I mean, "How embarrassing!" (Of course, the words always come back, with time. Though, on occasion, it may take months!)

So, as I may have a **Loss of Words** right in the middle of the spoken sentence, the same holds true for the written sentence. In writing this book, I may find myself leaving little hints about "the meaning of the word, I'm looking for," in hopes of recapturing it, while proofing. But, I may have to come back to *that place* many times, before the word reappears in my mind. That's alright; I'm constantly scanning for errors. (Not that I'd see them.)

I may read through a text several times, at different intervals, before I recognize the fact that I've used the wrong word, or that I've left out a word completely. You can see that this book is *Some Wonder*! So when you come across a mistake or lost word, (and you probably will), don't wonder, or wander. Just correct or fill-in the word of your choice. *Word Games* can be challenging and fun. Enjoy!

At work, I could not substitute typing for handwriting. You can just imagine how that went: i.e. … I'm writing a name with a capital "L" and it became a capital "Q." I couldn't figure out how to correct it. I could see that the loop of the "L" starts on the opposite side from the loop of the "Q," but I couldn't get my hand to do it. (Another faulty chip!) Speaking of "Q"; I would often reverse the circles on the letters B, D, P and Q. Like a child in school, I had to **mind my Ps and Qs**. It seems this computer, we call our brain, had dropped quite a few chips.

The delays in my reaction/reflexes, entered other areas of my life. My communication skills have become a shambles. Writing personal notes and letters became a nuisance. They looked sloppy. There would be attempts at erasures and white-outs or write-overs. I opted for the informal typewritten notes and letters, I had always considered inappropriate. Typing with correction ribbons, may not have been correct etiquette, but was legible. (Still, I make so many errors, correction tapes must be costing me a fortune.)

I knew there had been some physical injury to my right hand, from hitting the bed railing, when my arms shot-up from the SHOCK; but, we are talking *Neurological*, in this case. It was obvious, my hand-eye coordination was off. It was clear to see, one hand was slower than the other. I found this "Most Frustrating!" Trying to type anything, brought a multitude of errors. *Right* would show up as *rigth*. *Why* would become *Wyh* so often, my eyes had difficulty recognizing what, if anything, was wrong with it. (Another jig-saw puzzle.) I would go on looking for the solution; a way of getting-around the slow hand and returning to some sort of *Normal*. With any luck and the right therapy, I can conquer this. It still had not sunk in! You can not change Neurological Damage. The hand/eye coordination is off. **This is a permanent disability!** All of the therapy in the world, is not going to solve my typing problems. Of course, **THERE WAS NO CHANGE!**

When I evolved to the computer for my typing, corrections were easier and less expensive. (I'm no longer buying correction tapes.) Though I still make many mistakes, I find it easier to backspace, delete, and retype. With my slowed reaction time, it is faster than *Spell-Check*. Besides, *Spell-Check* could never unscramble this gobbledygook.

Sadly, the hands still will not work in unison. (And, never will.) I've had to **accept and adjust.** I know it would be a lot easier to do nothing, when there is no improvement, but **one must keep on keeping on.** This is one of those little things I will have to live with. We teach our Stroke Patients to talk, even if they aren't making sense. One hopes to build new pathways, by repetition. (As I had tried with my hand/eye coordination.) With some, this is possible. Some head injuries are worse than others, and this may not be possible. You can see where all traumatic head injuries would have differing symptoms, depending on the areas of their trauma. I can only speak of my disabilities, but they are small compared to those of many. I've found that **many will work hard at making a living, while others will have to work hard to simply make a life**. To whatever degree, you can count us among the "Challenged," but Determined.

* * * * * * *

* * * * * * *

COPING.....NOW.

My own methods of **coping with** the little disabilities of **day-to-day living** were as follows:

I could never remember if I had taken my daily pills. I had to make a **calendar graph** of my *medication, date*, and *time of day*. I have to refer back, to check if I've taken my pills. I am in a routine: I exercise, I eat breakfast and take my AM pills. At night: I watch the news, take my PM pills, shower, put a snack on top of the PM pills, and go to bed. If there is any variation in my routine, I may miss my medication. My husband will often remind me. He knows to check on me, if there is that change in my routine... telephone call, visitor, a load of clothes, a delivery, cup of tea, etc. The graph also comes in handy, when I am prescribed a few days of antibiotics. Doctors enjoy the running diary.

Lists are necessities! We can live without food for a few days, but not without our lists. Not only do I use a list for shopping, I also use a list of errands to run. (And, I'd better cross-off each errand; or, tomorrow I will run the same ones.) There will be lists for chores, for bills to mail, for calls to make with a list of subjects to cover, and a list for my doctor, of any problems or questions I may have, etc. I finally learned to <u>date the lists</u>, the day I made them. You may find one floating around in the glove compartment, a purse, or laundry basket. You will be able to throw it out, if it is out-dated; or, keep it for the day, if it is your current list. Let's tell the family right now: **Don't mess with our lists!** It took a lot of effort, in the first place; so, if we get excited about our lost lists, understand why. Put yourself in our place. Where would we be, without our lists? We may just buy a pair of shoes to match the new purse; shoes that, we had already bought two months before. Undated lists leave-you-open to a lot of useless investigative work.

There have been a few times, when I forgot I had a doctor's appointment, until I found the appointment card in my purse. I usually write it on my calendar, but I could forget. Just to double-check, I call the office to clarify the appointment, "My card reads Monday, June 23rd, but, I see June 23rd is on a Thursday. Is this a mistake? Should I come in on the 23rd, or on the Thursday following the 23rd? That would be the 26th." I'm told that I don't have a June appointment. That must have been a card from a previous year. Your appointment is for Thursday, July 12. ATTENTION RECEPTIONIST EVERYWHERE! Please include the year of our appointment. (Especially important in the office of a Neurologist.) Thanks.

Electronics are *Miserable Mysteries*, anyway; even for the non-challenged. The most nerve-calming contraption I've ever been blessed with, is the Over-The-Air TV Guide, which can automatically set-up and record your VCR, with the programs of your choice. You just check your on-screen menu, highlight the program of your choice, and push Record. Oh, Happy Day! Sure, I'm slow. (Remember, each day is a new day.) With my remote control, I must take it one-step-at-a-time, but I can accomplish the tasks.

I would like to say, I'm not as swift with electronics as I was before the SHOCK, but the truth is, I could never count on my recordings before the shock, either. Because each room had a different brand of VCR and TV with differing features, they required separate remote controls. (Do you see where I'm going here?) **That changed immediately!** We bought the same VCRs for all of the rooms. This is such a simple solution for the *Electronically Impaired*; but would have been much cheaper, if we had considered this, in the first place. This is something none of us think about. If one piece of equipment goes bad, we buy the best deal, with all of the latest *bells and whistles*. Sometimes, it might be easier to replace the *Electronically Impaired*. (Or, switch the *bells and whistles* to the kids room. They can handle anything electronic.) I'm still slow, but now I know how to handle it. **Man, talk about panic!** That was the day our TV went on-the-brink. I had to have it fixed ASAP. Disaster was averted, but how long will this 10-year-old TV last?!

As I talked of stumbling onto a solution, every now and then; this was a great help: While in a doctors' waiting room, I picked up a **Large Print Edition** of a magazine. As I begin to read, I noticed I was reading at a much faster pace than I had, since the SHOCK. Often, the problem with my hand/eye coordination, caused me to skip a line or re-read the same line, after coming to the end of a line of print. This was a real battle. With the A.D.S. and walking in a FOG, it was difficult for me to catch the meaning of the material being read. Perhaps the lines were too close together. I found that, with the Large Print, not only was the print bigger, but the line-spacing between each line was wider (separating the print more); allowing me to determine where the next line begin. Suddenly, there is no problem reading and comprehending the material. What a Blessing! (Too bad, it took ten years to stumble onto this!) **Therapists everywhere** should try the large print for their patients, who are having difficulty reading. It just might help!

It used to be, that I would put out the clothes I planned to wear tomorrow, the night before; but, if conditions changed, I was lost. If it turned cold or hot, if it rained or turned windy, it was back to the drawing board. The unexpected was always a bit overwhelming; it messes with my routine. I'm not so set on every outfit having to match, any more. I can wear most anything, the weather demands. If the outfit matches, that's a bonus, if it doesn't match, that's tough. Who cares? Really, who cares? They say that you come to a place in your life, when you learn that what others think, is not so important. First, to thine own self, be true. If you are happy doing what you think is right, then **that is right** for you. See! **Along the way, I am recapturing bits of the "Old Me."** Progress comes by baby steps. (I never cared what others thought!)

As we take hold of the positive things in our life, we forget the negative. We don't have time for the past, while looking to the future. Occasionally, everyone has a *down day*. When this happens, might I suggest you write about all of the good things that you have accomplished in your life, thus far. (Let's Count Our Blessings, so to speak.) Journaling good times, whets the appetite. It will lift your spirits and put you in a great mood. You realize, the simple things were the most memorable; not so much the expensive vacations, but the family times together. (Alright, if you have them, throw in those fabulous Decadently Expensive vacations to Distant Lands. But, those simple visits to Aunt Junes' house in Winter or Uncle Jerry's farm in Spring, may be more memorable.) The main thing is to **relive those beautiful times**. You may just write a line or two, but the memories that come flooding back to mind, are each a book unto themselves. Try it. You'll like it. It might *make-your-day*! A word or two is all you really need, to set you free to travel back to those days; and what a wonderful trip it will be. Oh, there may be a few times when things were not that great; like, learning to drive, your first ticket, a lost championship, lost love, etc.; but look at the knowledge gleaned from past experiences. See, the choice is ours. I tend to stick to the good times; don't want to ruin my run on *optimism*. It may just be that my past memories are all that I have, and they are precious. (Since I think in poetic terms; just overlook that.) Here are some samples of personal thoughts from my diary:

Taking my little hand in hers, as we walked along,
My Mother would sing to me, many wonderful songs.

Daddy read us stories, when we were still quite young.
Then, we would have to act them out, each and every one.

We had to grow up in the same County, as did Tom & Huck.
I would wish for every child, the same adventurous luck.

You see, I might have gone with few words: Moms' Songs, Dads' Stories, and Huck's Fun; but, look at all of the memories a few words can bring!

* * * * * * *

Socialize! Get out and about, as much as possible! Even if that means sucking in the fresh air from your back porch, do it with friends. You can phone a relative or friend, just to chat a bit. Or, go *on-line* for a quick chat, to keep in touch with friends and acquaintances. However, nothing beats socializing, face to face. Interactions, are so up-lifting. Do something that makes you put forth an effort, physically; even if it is just isometric exercises. These things help me and may help you. I know what you're thinking, **"Just what we need, suggestions from a Brain-Injured Person!"** Yes, that is exactly what we need; to help others with like problems.

I go on learning new revelations every day, but will they be there tomorrow? I was taught that you should learn something new everyday, no matter how small or insignificant it might seem. **Knowledge is the flower of growth, and wisdom the fruit thereof**. Sure, you say, "It is easy for you to learn something new each day; you can just learn the same thing you forgot yesterday." Perhaps, but it was mine for the day. And, who knows what is retained in this computer brain of mine? At least, I awaken each day, with eager anticipation, to see what it has in store. Every now and then, I amaze myself, with the information I spit out. It seems some things are retained, after all. It's encouraging, when they will emerge from some corner of the brain, when least expected. (Please! Don't interrupt my thought, or it's lost, again. Let me add to our conversation, on my own.) You never know. The information may be there for instant recall, one day. But, for now, let me wallow in a moment of new-found confidence. Meanwhile, let us enjoy what we have reclaimed. Look for the little everyday pleasures in your life. Look outward, not inward. **When you can find beauty in the bark of a tree, this is the proof, that you can finally see!**

Date/ AM / NOON / PM // / / DIARY / ACE / ASA

This is just a sample of a graph: You **always start with a date**, so you will know which day you are currently on. I date the whole sheet, before using. This way, you won't skip a day. List your morning pills under **AM,** your noon pills under **Noon**, and your afternoon or evening pills under **PM.**

I insert a couple of columns for emergency drugs that is **used rarely** (like Benadryl or Proventil). Then, I leave a good space for the **diary.** I just keep a running medical history of what unusual happenings occurred during that day. Most of the time, you won't have anything to write, but i.e. your legs are swollen, you have a cough, low blood sugar, high blood pressure, no sleep last night, nausea, etc. I add a couple of other columns for headache or pain medication; or, perhaps, antacid. It's your graph, change it to fit you.

I've arranged my calendar to fit regular bond paper size, and copy it front and back. (If you turn the paper over, then, turn it 180 degrees, it will be a continuous run.) Then I fold it in thirds and place it in a long envelope. This way, the calendar is a continuous record, ready to share with your doctors. (Or, for the EMT, **in case of an emergency**.) Keep a list of your current medications, allergies and this Medical

History sheet on your refrigerator or clipped to the inside of your front door. Keep neighbors and family apprized of this fact.

* * * * * * *

SPIN CYCLE, TOO.

What shall we do? What shall we do?
It seems it's time for Spin Cycle II.

What have they planned? I wish that we knew.
(Does Satin abound in these mischievous few?)

This ominous gang, with synchronous minds,
Come bearing untruths, of the bedeviling kinds.

The Time of Accountability had just passed.
So, what is to become of this? I ask.

The Statute of Limitation has just run-out.
Could that be what this is all about?

Sure, I'm a constant reminder of their wanton neglect.
Had the negative PR, given them belated regret?

Those hearing the story are simply aghast, wondering
"How many others had fallen prey, in the past."

"If they treat their employees with such disrespect,
What sort of care could their patients expect?"

"That's Food for Thought," some might say.
But, I say "It is just another day."

* * * * * * *

CHAPTER 9

SPIN CYCLE II

SPIN CYCLE II.....

Before starting ACT II of this PLAY, let me introduce you to the plot, it's Creators, and their character. Understand, the time for my chance to re-open this negligence case, had just passed. So, what could I expect? Certainly not compassion. Was I naïve enough to believe they were going to let me continue working? (I'm a constant reminder of their negligence!) They had let me keep working, to prove I was alright; so, I could still help pay-the-bills. Working was a struggle, but I had considered their willingness to work-with-me, a sign of compassion. With the past four years of slow but steady improvement, I should be able to do the job even better than I had been doing from the time of the Near-Electrocution. (If this FOG would just clear-up!) What are they doing to me? Had they really had my best interest in mind, or the interest of the Hospitals' Public Relations? What's the moral, here? Wait. I'm reminded of another time of compassion. The Nurses wanted Union representation; there would be a vote. The Hospital came up with all sorts of incentives and reasons why we should not go Union. "It would tarnish the dignity of the Profession. We need to work out all problems among ourselves. We want to work with you." (Gee, they had never done that before. I had seen nothing but indifference to everyone, who had ever had a problem.) To show how compassionate the Hospital was to our needs: "They understood that everyone was a *little short* on payday, so they were going to give us free lunches every payday;" insinuating we really didn't need Union interference. The Union vote failed. Our free lunches lasted two weeks, when it was decided that they were just too expensive to continue. Sure, we can readily see the moral here. *There is no such thing, as a free lunch.* But, **what's the moral, in my case?** I guess we can forget the bit about *Not looking a gift-horse* *in the mouth.* There was never a gift intended. Perhaps, *To trust no one*? I should stop being so gullible!

I was getting ready for my afternoon shift at work, when I received a phone call from my supervisor, informing me that I should not come in this afternoon. I asked if the census was down. "No, I am dismissing you." (She hadn't a clue.) I informed her that I was not currently serving on any committee. She stated, "No, I plan on dismissing you, permanently!" **I hadn't a clue!** With all of the good evaluations, nobody had mentioned a problem. **What a shock!** "Is something wrong?" I asked. "I think you know perfectly well, what is wrong," she replied. "I've set up a SKELLY Meeting in two weeks. You have the right to resign, without prejudice, before that time. If you choose to attend the SKELLY Meeting, I will dismiss you." (This sounds like a tape from *Mission Impossible*.) Never having had any experience with these meetings, I asked her what I would need to bring to the meeting. She reiterated that if I came to the meeting, I would be dismissed and lose the opportunity to resign.

There has to be some mistake. I'm a good nurse. Having been *"Called"* into the field, I loved my work, loved my patients, and my patients loved me. I'm thinking that we will be able to clear-up any misconceptions, at the meeting. I asked if she could give me a hint, as to what was wrong. "I don't like the way you treat your patients," she replied. I asked if she meant by that, the way I interacted with my patients or the quality of care? I received a curt, "Both." Dumb me! She probably couldn't have come up with that explanation on her own! Even so, she had never been so rude and hostile before. What's that all about? Three weeks before, she had given me five days off without pay, because of a disgruntled EMT. No specifics were given, but I had five days off. The Union said I should be paid for those days. "When was the last time you heard of an RN being evaluated by an EMT?" That never happens! (Sure, I'm being taken-advantage-of, but what can I do about it, in this FOG of confusion?!) My intuition tells me, that **I am being SET-UP**, for some reason, but I'm not grasping why. Oh well, I had a work injury to my right arm and shoulder; it was painful and needed a rest anyway. Of course, the Hospital should have been paying me for the injured shoulder! PLUS, my five days off; for harassment in the workplace. (I hope, you are not holding your breath!)

I notified the Union and they asked for copies of any complaints against me. The hospital would get the reports out… "right away." They must have had a hard time finding (or manufacturing) the complaints, because we didn't receive the copies until the day of the meeting…. I could come in early and take a look at the files involved…. not that I would be able to retain any of the information; and they certainly were not going to give us time to prepare. The Union representatives and I gathered in the Medical Records Room, to look over the complaints and the records involved. They gave me a copy of the first complaint. The Reps were not surprised in the least, when they heard me laugh. (I still laugh, to this day.) I was being portrayed as the worse person that had ever walked the face of the earth, while the girl writing the report, was "walking on water." The contrast was just too much!! What a laugh! About the only truth to her diatribe, was at the end: "And so, this is my story." And, a fine one it was. Was her story manufactured? Though it was insignificant, it contained one item that could have only been known, had she had access to my personnel files. You have to feel that the poor girl has a conscious somewhere, because of the horrible thing **she** had said to a patient, was now being attributed to me. At least, she had realized that her behavior had been inappropriate. (See, I should have been *writing-up* her behavior? Talking to the supervisor had done nothing.) At any rate, this will all come out in the meeting. I'm not overly concerned. Everything will be straightened out, then. If you tell the truth, the truth will set you free.

Or…maybe not… The meeting was a farce. You could see the famous jaw-set of determination. Minds were made-up, beforehand. This was only a facade of justice. Whatever it takes to get rid of me, they were going to do. With some difficulty, they scarcely pretended to show interest in anything we had to say. But, with my adamant denials and the Unions protest, they would set another SKELLY Meeting. In the mean time, the Supervisor would get us copies of the "dozen or so complaints" she had stored in her own personal Departmental Files. **I still don't understand. Help me, here. If my supervisor had all of these many complaints, why hadn't she discussed them, during my evaluations? Isn't a supervisor supposed to discuss problems, so they will be resolved? That sounds like *dereliction of duty* to me!** (Maybe they hadn't counted on a second meeting.) The Union asked for a face-to-face meeting with my accusers. The request would be taken into consideration. (I'm really not naïve, just in a FOG!)

We would await the copies of the many Departmental Complaints. In the meantime, I prepared a *line-item veto* of the many accusations of the first girl. I'm ready. I could hardly wait to confront her and the RN: who had claimed that she had to go into one of my rooms and tell me that my patient was having PVCs; "Even though, I was standing right there, I hadn't recognized the problem." I'm sure the whole world is going to believe this girl! I'm current on all of the major certificates (ERN, BCLS, ACLS, and PALS) and she chooses the most obvious dysrhythmia. Even someone watching "Chicago Hope" or "ER" would recognize possible PVCs. (In reality, I was across the hall, cleaning a room, after sending that patient to surgery. I had been monitoring my sleeping patient on the overhead monitors above the Nurses Station. We were awaiting the results of his Digoxin Level.) Like many others, she really hadn't any idea of how Short Term Memory worked. She was another person who thought that every situation, would be lost in an instant. Wouldn't she wonder how I kept up with all of my certifications? Oh, yeah! That's right! But, of course she wouldn't. i.e. I'm reminded of the time we were taking a Trauma Core Course together. I had this horrible headache with burning red eyes, so I took a gram of acetaminophen every four hours. We were both wondering how we did on the tests, as we went to have them checked. She went in first, and when she came out she said I had nothing to worry about. The woman had let her change-back five of her answers, so she would pass. (Well, they certainly were laid-back and cooperative. That was encouraging. My eyes burned so much, I could hardly see; but, I'm pretty sure I had passed the test anyway. It probably would not be the usual high grade, but I'll take what I can get, in this condition.) I went in for my results. The woman berated me for making such a low score. "I should have scored in the nineties!" In her estimation, "Seventy-eight is a poor score, but it is still passing." I guess this nurse knew how they played the game, for her. I'm here to tell her, they did not play the game the same for everyone. And the horrible headache? At 4:00 PM, as I ran past the ER to take another gram of acetaminophen, I checked my temperature. It was 104.0 degrees. (Is it any wonder I forgot to turn my patient over, during the clinical part of the test? I guess not. It turned out, that I had a horrible bladder infection.) ☺ So, why her blatant lies? Could it be guilt or just plain ignorance? I don't know. Perhaps, a little of both.

This was the same *"brilliant nurse"* who did our scheduling. I was told that she often scheduled herself for *doubling back.* If you doubled back two shifts in the same day, you could receive double-time pay. If she was too tired to do the double, she would ask one of we "On-Call" nurses to work in her place. We were not always available. This had been one of those days. She came into the Report Room, letting us know that she was doubling back and she was really too tired to work. For her assignment, she would be taking "Charge" tonight, and she didn't want anyone to disturb her unless it was an absolute emergency; she would be in the doctors lounge, sleeping! We saw little of her the entire shift, but she had to come out and give a report to the on-coming shift at eleven o'clock. Not a happy camper! What makes some people so mean? Who knows? They just seem to be angry and unhappy people. Perhaps, just over-worked; a case of "burnout."

Imagine this little old man of Near Eastern decent, in the ER with bradycardia; and he decided to take a nap, while awaiting laboratory results. Can you even begin to imagine how he might react, if he had some "*screaming mamie*" come to the foot of his bed and awaken him from a sound sleep?! She is screeching, "Oh, my God! This guy is having bradycardia! (But what does he know? It's the same thing he came into the ER with. She sounded as if he was at Deaths' Door.) "Now, he is having PVCs. Get the doctor in here! What do you know about this mans' history?" The same thing she might have known, had she not been in the doctors' lounge, all night. ***("What's that mean? Am I going? Why is she screaming? I feel okay, but she must see something.")*** Under these circumstances, he just might be expected to have a PVC or two. She is lucky she hadn't killed him! He hadn't had a PVC before she came into his room, and he never had another PVC for the rest of his stay in the hospital… for observation. Yes, *stay for observation*! This nutty nurse, had just cost the taxpayers more money. (I'm from Missouri, so, "Show me." I often wondered <u>if</u> and <u>where</u> this girl had attended nursing school?) Of course, she also thought the man was cyanotic; even though, his O2 saturation remained 100%. (And the SKELLY SKIT wanted to know why I hadn't charted the changes in the patients condition. Well, maybe because… <u>There were no changes</u>?!) If he was cyanotic, so was the rest of his family. My little man was doing fine. She had made a fool of herself, big time. No amount of C.Y.A. was going to change the fact that she had nearly scared the patient to death. I have never known a *real nurse* who would risk a patients well-being, especially in an emergency, by loud scare tactics.... Thinking somehow, this makes you look important? It makes you look like an idiot. (Which, of course, you are.) Try to act like a real Nurse!

Please, learn the art of gentle persuasion, while taking decisive actions. Speak calmly, to calm a patient. His life often depends on his cooperation. He will only cooperate if he feels he is in the hands of competent, compassionate people. Remember your patient is right there; speak to him and let him know what you are doing. (Don't scream past him, as if he were just a piece of furniture.) As others come into the room to help, keep the calm communication going. There is seldom a reason for raising your voice. We can stop verbal abuse; and, we can stop the patients' uncertainty about his condition, with quiet respect. If tests are needed to determine his condition, let him know.

Another nurse stated, "As an experienced ER Nurse (Experienced? New!), according to what the first girl said had happened (CYA, meaning: Covering Your Asterisk), I do not feel this nurse competent to work a busy ER." So this was the big third complaint against me! (Hearsay?) These two had been sent home early one evening, due to low census. The EMT said she wasn't going home... they could just find someone else. She had car-pooled and didn't have a way home. "You can just send Joel home." She was informed that Joel had just started his shift and no one was sending him home. She could hang around, if she wanted to, but she would be clocking-out at 10:00. I'm not sure this girl had ever been told "NO" before. (This must have made her a *disgruntled EMT*.) The "experienced" nurse was the other one chosen to go home early. Perhaps they could go home together, since they lived in the same city. I'm saying nothing... I lived in the same city, also; but I'm not about to take her home in my car. She was rude and mouthy to me at work, I sure wasn't going to put up with her mouth for an hour-drive home! Stupid, I'm not! Well, maybe. It did give them time to dream up a beautiful story together. A whole hour-drive home! At least, the *experienced nurse* was smart enough to keep her complaint "hearsay;" sure protection from a lawsuit. Though, I'm sure the EMT was not smart enough to compose her story without help; she had left herself wide open. Still, she was good at one story. One wonders if the driver was aware of the fine story the EMT was telling about her. We certainly learned more than any of us needed to know about her personal life. That is why it is called personal; it belongs to that person.

Every now and then, we need to step back and see, that we are all God's children. We are created by the MASTER Potter, from the same lump of clay; every one of us a MASTERpiece. And, GOD does not make mistakes. HIS children, however? That's an on-going story. Oh, well. ☺

We would await the supervisor's many *Personal* Departmental Complaints. (Once again, Genius, why wasn't I informed of such things??) I had prepared that *line-item veto* of the accusations of the first girl. Boy, I was ready! Just wait until we meet, **face-to-face!** IT NEVER HAPPENED! We came to the next SKELLY Meeting prepared, but they had taken our request into consideration and felt it was not necessary. (Same jaw-set noted.) And the dozen or so Departmental Complaints?? There were none. (Ah, so that is why I had not heard of the Personal Departmental Complaints before! Sounds like more C.Y.A.) When the Union stated that they had not received copies of the other complaints, they were told that we had received all of the complaints. "You mean the original three?" "That is correct. You have received all of the complaints." (None of these people will ever be mistaken for Rocket Scientist! What if there is a second SKELLY Meeting? Maybe they shouldn't lie on the first tape.) I think, someone had "called-their-bluff." How many others had been railroaded, in the same Game of Chance?

A "Patients' Privacy" prevents us from interviewing the patients for the truth. I told my husband that we could just take polygraph tests, to determine who was telling the truth. In my *FOG,* I was serious! He reminded me that polygraphs were only used in murder trials, and other *life and death* situations - not in *life-changing* situations. (This was very serious to me. The murder of my reputation!) We could have pushed this thing, even though the complaints were worded in such a way, that it would have been a "She said," "No, she said," situation. We could tell that this was all a farce, but the Union said, "If a Company wants to get rid of you, there is nothing you can do about it." The Union was well aware of the fact that I had no intention of continuing to work with these liars, anyway… not even for the two weeks they suggested, so I could resign. We could see the light coming down the tracks… I was being **RAILROADED!** I made them fire me. I was again offered a chance to resign without prejudice. (They could only hope that I would go for their little plan.) I refused. So, when you look back at my history and say, "Gee, she was fired!" You might be thinking, in reality, **"No! She fired them!"** I had done nothing wrong and they knew that! I had been lied to and lied about. To accept that behavior, was to condone it. My principles are too high for that. (They should have known that, too!) Principles are not for sale. If you haven't principles, what have you? A person must do what they feel is right. **(And, the morals, in this case? They have none!)** They might, also, guess… I would not be finding another job anytime soon. After four years of slow, but gradual improvement, I am suddenly incompetent! Amazing! (Gee, I was very competent, while the Company was trying to prove that I was well enough to work.) Never mind my trying to find the Med-Room or the X-Ray Department in a different hospital. (Remember, I already knew where everything was in this hospital, before the Near-Electrocution.) Presently, with the on-going *Short Term Memory Loss*, how would I find my way around, at a new place of employment?

Effective FORCED RETIREMENT !!

It was time. I was amazed at how easy it was for me to walk away. Talk about shaking the dirt from your sandals and walking away… I never looked back. As I walk away, I feel freed. It is one of those times of peace that surpasses human understanding. It has become the past! More importantly now is, when will the next opportunity present itself, when I can once again help my fellow man? I will need to wait and be patient. I've always found that *when one door closes, another opens.*

I received unemployment; and though I had always hoped to work until I was seventy, I had to go on Social Security Disability. Early retirement! Benefits would be, but a fraction of what I would have received at the age of seventy. **(Hey, I've been robbed of my retirement!)** When I talked to Social Security about retiring early, they asked if I shouldn't take disability. To show how foggy things were for me; I was not in a wheelchair, so I hadn't considered myself *disabled.* I was still in denial. I just wouldn't use that *word*, when referring to myself. I guess it was a matter of pride …... something about taking a hand-out. To convince me, the interviewer had to give me several examples of others who were disabled, yet not confined to wheelchairs. There are other head injuries, with a variety of deficits; amnesia, disorientation, seizures, and other mental problems. How about Personality Disorders, Alzheimer's, A.D.S., etc.? (Sure, like Attention Deficit; or maybe, Short Term Memory Loss?) He is right, of course. Disability happens in many forms. He told me that I could take temporary disability and if I got better, we could change it. He could readily see, that it was going to take a while for me to accept this reality. Who would have guessed?

There is a reason for everything. I would see this, eventually. I had never really found time to relax, during this entire episode; never allowed myself to linger on the tragedy, only the progress. In my confusion, I was fighting hard to hold on to my illusion of normalcy; trying to convince others, I would be alright, given time. For now, I need to take some time to just relax and *"smell the roses."* Forget the work schedule! (Of course, It would have been much easier, with Workers' Compensation; I would not have had to worry about getting enough work to help pay the bills. These people are truly unconscionable, for the fraud they perpetrate on innocent victims!) The only thing I need right now, is to work on getting stronger and healthier. Despite the roadblocks, I can do this! Just being able to slow down and relax, gives me new insight. Little by little, I am recapturing bits of reality. It's a beautiful world!

* * * * * * *

When I look back at my frailties, I see that I could *dish-the-dirt* with the best (or worst) of them. Though I managed to keep the thoughts to myself, I did have the thoughts; proving base instincts. At least, I kept it real. Did it make me feel better? Not really; it is just another embarrassing part of my past. It was that child-like behavior, in an adult, *acting-out*. Why would you waste so much time, on something like that? Lack of control, thanks to the decreased inhibition. I will need to fill my time with positive reinforcement, in order to find the real me. I'm refusing to give-in to that lack of control.

* * * * * * *

Mystery, Intrigue, Deceit and the Will to Survive.

You have learned the ***mystery*** of the Living Dead, as well as many other mysteries. Then, there is the ***intrigue*** of human nature, finding the foibles of the weakened, with the ***deceit*** that takes advantage, while seeking to destroy. (Though it doesn't make it right, wild animals do the same.) That ***will to survive?*** Finding a way to overcome the stumbling blocks, outwit the nitwits, and out-maneuver their inner-child mentality.

In order to **solve** any mystery, you have to face the facts: Some things can never change. Many of my symptoms from the burn of the current, will remain a mystery. While some have improved, many remain the same, and some may be yet to come. I have accepted these truths. I don't know what the future holds for me. Let's face it, nobody really knows what the future holds. I guess that makes me normal, when you look at this reality. There are definite variables. We have natural disasters, like: lightening strikes or floods; and calamities, like: falling off of your bicycle into a rose bush, or tripping over an extension cord and taking a bite of grass. (Well, they are natural calamities to you. You certainly are not *clumsy* or *unbalanced.*) Then, we have the unexpected Human Nature disasters.

You hope to ***dissolve*** the treachery of deceit and intrigue, by disclosing the culprits. Just as those who commit murder, feel they will never be caught; those who seek to murder a reputation, feel they are so clever, that they too, will never be caught in their webs of lies and deceit. If they could only see themselves as others see them! They fool no one but themselves. Lies never go away; you cannot take them back. They will always come back to bite you, whether you care or not. (Many don't really care. It is the only excitement they find in their lives.)

So, you absolve the sociopathic minds, who live the lives of deceit, daily; accepting these people for who they are – not who you wish they could be. When you learn to "Consider the Source," nothing surprises you, nor overwhelms you. These are the days we live in. **Resolve**, this will not change your life. You choose your friends wisely; those who exude joy and happiness. Fun and peace are priceless. At the same time, we know that it takes all kinds to make this old world. Who said, "What a boring place this old world would be, if everyone in it, were exactly like me?" (I don't know who said it, but I've been using it for years. Thanks.) I still choose to see the best in people.

CHAPTER 10

A REASON FOR STUBBORN PERSEVERANCE

A REASON FOR STUBBORN PERSEVERANCE...

Strangely enough, I am still great with numbers. I can stand in line at the store and figure my items (with the taxes) to the penny, by the time I get to the register. With all of this difficulty, I can keep the checkbook and do the taxes. No problem with numbers. I wish it were so easy with this book. The anatomy of this *challenged writer* might be like this: Time is of the essence. I must finish a complete chapter in one day. Tomorrow is another day and I will have forgotten what I've written today. At first, this was all impossible. I would dredge the material from the notes I maintained for my neurologist, regarding my progress. Then, I have to put bits and pieces together, in some sort of order that would be understood. Not an easy task, in a confused and intimidated state. **Why can't I remember?** These things happened to me. I would have to look back at the previous chapter to see if I was using the *first person* or coming from the point of an *on-looker.* (The **Short Term Memory** problem.) Finally, I've learned that only I could tell this story. That doesn't mean that I won't find LIKE chapters... meaning that I had already written about the subject before. (It's encouraging, to some extent. That computer brain of mine must be retaining something.)

I'm typing about one subject, when thoughts drift; and I am typing about another subject. (That's **Attention Deficit.**) I will find complete paragraphs, in two different works, that are word-for-word. Something is up there; just not available for voluntary instant recall. You weed-out and keep the version you like best. Since the same subjects might appear in two different chapters, I must weed them, also. Finally, I came up with a solution to that problem... I put a list of contents on the front of each chapter. I may get somewhere, after all; but, it will take time. Forgive me if the subjects seem scattered, I'm doing the best I can. (We are back to those indispensable lists again. Without them, this book is destined to become an *unfinished symphony.* I have to keep that sense of humor.)

I guess this would be that *"whole other story"* in *"another chapter"* I wrote about. There are many things we may not have experienced, back in our "normal life," which would just bring added confusion, after our disaster. In those days, before the crisis, no one *pulled the wool over our eyes.* Now, <u>YOU WILL BE</u> <u>taken-advantage-of</u>. Expect it and have an advocate at your side. Especially, when a deposition interviewer has *difficulty comprehending* the many doctors reports, and he is there *to verify* medical information from the injured party. (Their lawyer kept drilling me on things I had no recollection of. Hello! Is anybody there? I do have Short Term Memory!)

Of course, it would be ten or eleven years later, before I could try to decipher what the many reports were saying. I figured I would, at least, try to understand the many papers involved with this incident. It would be a real eye-opener, to see how masterfully the Hospitals' lawyer muddied the playing field, confused and manipulated some doctors into changing their minds about their original reports. This was **not** a matter of **ignorance after all**, but **rather, a concerted effort to defraud**; a matter of *doing business*, effectively. If that demands lies and manipulation, so be it. It seems various doctors were given selective pieces of information, only. An unscrupulous Corporation can always find unscrupulous cohorts. <u>Have an advocate</u>, to watch out for your rights.

Just as the wild beast seeks the weakest of the herd to attack, so too, will the lead Jackal of the pack, seek to destroy the disabled. *He is Selling his soul to the Devil, so to speak. Of course, his master is the Corporation he represents.* "Hey, it's just a job and someone has to do it." *Or, do they?*

Sure, I was in a state of confusion and couldn't understand why I was not awarded Workers Compensation for such a serious injury as the **Near-Electrocution,** when they gave me a small sum for my Tennis Elbows. It just so happened that I had good records; thanks to the logs I was instructed to keep, regarding my progress or any new problems. Maybe the logs were too thorough! They would be misused. I would come to see, in writing, and understand the reason for the compensation discrepancy, in due time.

I'll give a few examples of how the depositions work. Corporations' Insurance Company reads the doctors' reports, and then sends their lawyer out to take a deposition, to see if the doctors were aware of "such and such." *"I don't want to influence you, but their are a couple of things I needed to check."*

The woman, for whatever reason, felt compelled to keep a diary of various complaints. (Maybe, because of the **SHORT TERM MEMORY.**) *She really didn't mention the trigger finger for weeks. I have tons of records here. You are free to go through them, but I can assure you, it was weeks.*

The doctor being interviewed said, "I don't think I've seen those records before."

The interviewer again: *"They're kind of interspersed ...they weren't exactly in chronological order.* (**Of course, my Medical Logs were in order, and stapled in order**.) *But what I want to point out is this: I will assert to you- and I'll leave these with you in case you want to review them for any reason. But I will ask you to assume that when you read through these, the first notation about any problem with the knuckle, is weeks later."*

The doctor being interviewed (let's call him M) was sticking with his diagnosis and prognosis all along; through such statements as *"I'm going to ask you to assume. Would that alter your opinion?* May I see those notes you just read to me? *I got tons of them. I will guarantee.* I don't remember seeing these records. *They were interspersed in a funny place in one of the sets of medical records.* (He must have shuffled them like a deck of cards, showing different doctors, just what he wanted them to see.) Maybe I missed them. **(CREATED SELF-DOUBT.)** *Let's see. I'm pretty sure you have had these records, but I wouldn't be surprised if you missed them.*

M: Can we go off the record for a second? The way this is written suggest that these symptoms had been going on for some time, but obviously with somebody who is writing absolutely day by day, what looks like everything that bothers her, it's hard to say that it's really been present since November of 1991. (**BINGO! Mission Accomplished?**)

I don't want you to be misled. She did complain about numbness of both hands, at the time. The grip strength seemed to be normal. (Did they forget to mention the flexion deformity? No, the manipulator chooses only the right subjects, for his manipulation.)

M: **A trigger finger can be caused by anything that you would get a swelling around the flexor tendons. I would say that the trigger finger was indeed caused by the injury of November, 1991. It doesn't sound like something that just came on all at once. It is written like it was something that was already there.** (I'm proud of this doctor. He is not going to have the wool pulled over his eyes!) **But** I suspect with this lady's compulsiveness of writing day by day by day all of her symptoms, if she had been bothered by her trigger finger, she would have mentioned it somewhere earlier. **NOW, MISSION ACCOMPLISHED!)** You can't blame this doctor. He was honest, but had an ***accomplished adversary***. This interviewer had played the **"crackpot" hypochondriac** card. No one would know about the months we spent trying to stop the tachycardia, chest pain, and weakness. Somehow, these seemed more crucial to record, at that time.

I'm beginning to understand the discrepancies in the reports. I'm sure the main playing card to all of the innocent participants in my case; was trumped with a "Hypochondriac Joker." It may not be Poker, but everyone plays games. (A nice way of saying fraud and deceit; as if there is a nice way!)

On to our ***Preferred Provider:*** We were amazed at the "filler" he included in his report. I feel sorry for **whoever it was,** that had multiple Kaiser Hospital visits, dating from 1962 and 1982. It was not me! (I would like to see him produce those reports, if they really do exist.) I guess I was just too busy traveling the World, Scuba Diving, and flying airplanes; but, of course, *Time flies, when you're having so darn much fun.* I did manage to fit in another baby however, during that time. We also raised our children, and I went back to college, while working my job. I'd say I had a pretty full schedule. We'll give him that *benefit of a doubt*, and say it was probably someone else's chart. (I would notice, at this time, that they had been using my **wrong first name**, for all of these years. I'm sure that complicated matters.) Forget the benefit of a doubt! The next paragraph of his report was as follows: 'Office notes from 1976 through 1986, signature unintelligible, were noted.' (Well, there you go. That is certainly enough to deny compensation!) I would like to see that report, also. What can I say? Was the good doctor, *"doctoring"* his reports? Since my car had been hit in a couple of accidents over the years, he automatically padded his report, by **assuming two previous Whiplashes** for me. DIDN'T HAPPEN!! You know what they say about assuming anything. But, if you are already an.....

In February of 1993, about 14 months after my Near Electrocution, the Hospital arranged for a deposition, for Workers Compensation. (I'm still in that Fog of confusion, which would last for six years.) I feel, it was an effort to ***strike fast, before she knows what's going on***. Even so, I can't believe these people put me through this deposition, in my condition! They were fully aware of their negligence and my inability to find answers to their questions; that is why they had copies of my medical logs. I am slow mentally; that slow assimilation of material, along with the Short Term Memory. The Hand/Eye coordination is "off," making reading and searching for written material a slow, frustrating process. Their report from the Neuropsychologist would verify these problems. There should be no limit on reopening a Workers' Comp case of a disabled person; especially, when they have been fraudulently ***taken-advantage-of***. (I was still in my naïve years.) As I read through the deposition ten years later, I found it as confusing as it would have been back then; however, I can readily see glaring mistakes today! Still, I am helpless to correct the errors of the past. Ah, if only I had the ability to read, comprehend, and make decisions for instant action, as I once had; but, that would not be my reality.

My lawyer (You know, the one who would lend his name to my requests for mileage reimbursement and the one who had me sign for dismissal of any compensation from the Near-Electrocution? That one.) and the interviewers were having a great time. Aside from the Hidden Indians, they couldn't get over a gynecologist named Pushpa; envisioning women in childbirth, hearing "pushpa, pushpa, pushpa." You could tell, they were not taking this deposition seriously. On top of my disabilities, I had not had a good nights' sleep for the past two nights, thanks to that "Sunburn" feeling across my back. The "Sunburn" was very uncomfortable; I couldn't find a comfortable position, for sleeping. This made it very easy for the interviewer to slide in the wrong answers, where they needed them. i.e. in one incident, a wheelchair injured my right ring finger. He had me tell him which finger it was, a couple of different times; then said, *So, the wheelchair hurt your right middle finger, right?* My answer? "Correct." He referred to it again, as he went over his list… *oh, that's the right hand; I believe the middle finger that was hurt by the wheelchair.* **(That would discredit the injury to my right middle finger,** when it hit the bedrail, as my hands flew over my head, during the SHOCK. Just like the **whiplash** episode above, was meant to discredit my present **neck pain** with occasional numb hands.) I could never have followed any of this, back then. I'm not sure I could, today. He need not have worked so hard. He went on playing "mix and match" with doctors names, cities, hospitals, dates, health problems or incidents, times off from work, and etc. It is so evident, he is manipulating this whole session.

After one break, the interviewer said, *"Now, where were we?"* My lawyer said that the next thing he had on his list was the **Tachycardia**. (Strange, they never got back to the Tachycardia; and I certainly could not be expected to remember.)

No, I want to talk about a left lung injury in 1974, from pulmonary emboli.

Then, he covered the bronchitis I had in 1985; the coughing caused costochondritis. Maybe these two instances were what caused **the numbness under my ribcage**, 15-25 years later. (Maybe that would discredit the fact that I have no sensation under the ribcage or in the abdomen. Nah! I don't think so. I don't know anyone that dumb.)

It seems he purposely intertwined two instances of allergic reactions to IVP Dyes; one happened in about 1962, and the other a few years before my SHOCK. In the first episode, I had to be checked by a Neurologist. In the second episode, I incurred a Prolapsed Mitral Valve. I survived both episodes without residual effects. Even, the prolapsed valve resolved itself. (So, would that discredit any new **Brain Injuries** and **Heart Conditions** associated with the Near Electrocution? Not really!) As we read through the many doctors' records and depositions, we could see the conspiracy; every symptom of the Near Electrocution had to be discredited, no matter what it took. The whole incident had to disappear; as if it had never even existed. This is why so much effort was put into erasing the facts; yet, other minor injuries were given a spotlight. The hospital was seeking noble credibility. **This Hospital was not going to take responsibility for their negligence!!**

Is it really our fault? Oh No! Don't put that on me! What do we think of these injustices? Most of us feel helpless. Because we do nothing, the fraud grows year after year. It is not something new. How many years has it been since the Hostile Corporate take-overs; where a Corporation would see a struggling business with a huge pension fund. They would buy the business at a discounted price and abscond with the pension funds. How about a CEO who is hired to "turn-around" a fledging airline? While siphoning-off Company assets to his own "Holding Company," grabbing a *Golden Parachute*, after taking the Airline into bankruptcy. But, you say, how could these things happen to the retirees; and how about all of the people who lost their jobs?! The stockholders were left *holding the bag*?! Where is our compassion?! We have the compassion, but still, we feel helpless. Aren't we sick of hearing, "It may be immoral, but not illegal?" We know that they are just "playing games" with the Justice System. Why don't we start our protest, by calling it like it is? They are liars, thieves, embezzlers, cheaters, greedy, fraudulent, crooks, etc. **How Unpatriotic Would You Be**, to create an "off-shore" bank account, to avoid paying taxes to the Country that helped you succeed? We could have no deficits, if everyone pulled their fair share. *It may be immoral, but not illegal*!! We have to stop making them sound so benign. Only then, will we hold them accountable. ***Playing Games*, indeed!**

This was just a sampling of the tools of fraud. If you cannot help your situation, due to your disability, don't hurt your situation by trying to handle things you are not capable of. It is difficult, assigning someone else a part of your power. We, the *Disabled*, are already fighting to regain our power; those things we can no longer do for ourselves.

With Brain Injuries, we may not understand the degree of our damage. Some of us think that we are quite capable of taking charge of our lives. This is only an illusion. With our foggy reality: We could bathe and dress ourselves. We could feed ourselves. I could drive my car. We can talk to our friends and family, play with the dog, grocery shop (of sorts), get the mail, ride the bus, play soccer, or bake some cookies, do your homework, or even work a job. ***In reality*, *we are*** just ***learning to cope*** with our disabilities. (I would still rather fight for futile recovery, than to sit there with no hope. Keep focused on the things you can do, and work with hope and take a chance on improvement in the future. We never know what miracles await around the bend.)

Keeping up with my Certifications for work, took some ingenuity. With the loss of my Hand/Eye coordination, the overhead projected EKG strips were not sufficient. I could not see the whole strip, at once. I was given actual strips, to use for the tests. That worked. After all, it is the actual strips that we measure, in the end. I wonder how many students with Hand/Eye disabilities (This is where the eye sees, but the brain is slow to recognize the information and turn it into a reaction.) are asked to follow Overhead Projected material. Add Attention Deficit to the equation, and the student is really lost. Had he seen and comprehended the whole concept, on the overhead? (I know how that works… by the time you get to the end of the sentence, you may have forgotten the first of the sentence.) **Teachers**, you may well have to depend on individual books and materials, for the brain injured student. Remember, their disability need not be massive, to be a *stumbling block.* The Large Letter Editions of books are not just for the people with poor eyesight. I found them much easier for me to read and comprehend, because I was not losing my lines or repeating the same lines over again. The print has enough room between lines, to let me see which line is next. This really speeded my reading back to normal. It's worth a try.

(Reaction time and memory still won't cooperate, but I can read faster.) Maybe it's false confidence, but I do feel more confident with each success.

Since I could not read and comprehend as quickly as before, I was given a Minnesota IQ test to take home and finish… no hurry, I had a week. (Well, it's not like I could look back and change my answers; I go to sleep, and the next morning is that *New Day* dawning. I have already forgotten yesterday.) I do wish I knew what I put on that test, to make the Doctor believe I did so well, "to make herself look good." I do grasp a significant piece of material from some of the doctors reports, that will tell me what part of the brain is involved with my disabilities, but I'm not sure it sinks in yet. So the **conspicuously low psychomotor speeds**, means what? (I know I am slow, mentally.) The **discrepancy between my verbal and visual memory is significant**, whatever that means. (I would guess that has something to do with my Hand/Eye coordination being "off.") I can not go into specific reasons, now. I am still working with the results. I really don't need a medical name for my problems (the symptoms are ever-present), but it is good to see them, in writing. Some people really are aware of the reasons for these disabilities. This gives us hope that someone is working on alleviating, or curing, the symptoms. Even new coping mechanisms, will help make our lives easier.

Though, I was not capable of giving a deposition, "That's okay." I was assured I wouldn't have to recall *current events*. After all, I had given them the history of my progress; the medical logs, and the pre-SHOCK medical records. They just needed me there to verify that they understood the records appropriately. (Should I have believed that? That was in the days, when I believed all adults told the truth.) I should not have been put through a deposition. When I look at how the names, times, places, dates, and incidents were shuffled, I'm very disappointed in the purposeful deception and fraud, performed against me, by the Hospital and their representative. The sad fact is, there are many that have, and will be, fraudulently denied justice. I'm sure we all know someone who has injuries from some work-related accident, who are being ignored. If you have received a disabling brain injury, you will be defrauded. Take precautions, and take a friend. You really need a trusted friend or relative at your side for each doctors visit, deposition, interview, and etc., to stay-on-top of the facts. (All of my close friends and relatives were in a distant State. I had no one, except my husband; and he was working a full-time job. There were times when he had to take-off work for some of my medical tests, but using his vacation time on my care, seemed degrading to me; though, he never thought it a burden.) You know that it is the Culprits dream, to find a brain-injured victim who has no family to answer to. It's a shame these people can not be trusted, when it comes to brain injuries; or, for that matter, any disabled person. Be sure to have someone with you, to keep them honest. **AS IF !!**

I was so tempted to divulge the name of the scoundrel working for the Hospital, but then, we know all about Peters Principle. (Most of the people involved in this fraud, got where they are today, through Peters Principle.) You know there are other unscrupulous Corporations, who would pay *this scoundrel* twice as much, to get a proficient liar like him, to come work for them. (It seems that Fraud and Deceit are currently "In.") It takes someone thoroughly unprincipled, to do this job. Forget it! Let him make his mark, right there! The sad thing is, you know that the Hospital and the other liars, are very proud of their work. Too bad! They are missing the pride of a job well done, while contributing to society. Then again, I'm sure, some are happy with their low self-esteem, and quite contented with being a second-class citizen. Some seem to revel in it.

Having said it all, I've left nothing to the imagination. There are no great secrets left untold about my experience. I hope we have helped you to be aware of some of the pitfalls you may encounter. Don't be completely naïve. My husband and I were both too trusting. We thought that the Company, Insurance Representatives, Lawyers, and Courts were there to help the disabled. My husband felt confident enough in the abilities of these folks, he didn't have a second thought about their integrity; thinking they would only do the very best to see that I was *taken care of* appropriately. (No! *Not* to be *Ruined* or *Eradicated*!) So, when I say the many reports were eye-openers for us, I meant the both of us. Still, the average God-fearing Americans, can be trusted; they strive to do the right thing. Because of this, we will continue trusting in the best in people.... But, perhaps, with a little more caution. Maybe we'll recognize the "fish stories" for what they are, and enjoy the moment. Meanwhile, like my brother would say, "Consider the Source."

Before the **C**risis, I could have written this book in three months. Nothing really makes sense anymore. Life is in slow-motion. I have that darn "Lag Time." I struggle with this book for the others who are suffering from the same condition. Not so much for the victims, as for the family and friends who will read and comprehend the loneliness we feel. It's rough feeling that nobody can possibly understand what is going on. I will try to enlighten: For me, the mental disabilities were worse than my physical problems. I looked pretty normal. I had no charred flesh hanging from my bones, so everyone surmised I was alright. People have a hard time accepting neurological problems, when one looks so physically normal. If they have the time, those in daily contact, can readily see the decreased concentration, the slowed reaction time, and that *"Doe caught in the headlight"* syndrome. The tiny spatter burns on both arms would heal. The hole burned through the mucous membrane of my nasal septum would eventually grow back. (Meanwhile, it looked like I had a pearl in one side of my nose.) My nerve pathways have been cooked. Only time would tell which pathways would mend and which would retain scars. Scars, like ruts on an old country road, are mysteries; you can never see or ascertain how deep they go. I would get the feelings back in my hands; though, that right middle finger injury turned into a Trigger Finger. Holding my fingers straight, I could type. Even with all of the mistakes my typing entails,

I am able to communicate by letter. Meanwhile, gripping a pencil is painful and tiring. Needless to say, my handwriting is terrible. Flossing took courage. Reaching for the back teeth on the right, you knew the finger would go out-of-joint. That is very painful. The feelings never returned under my ribcage, to my abdomen, or nostrils and back of throat. It would be Six Years after the Near-Electrocution, before the FOG lifted. **(I AM SO GRATEFUL!!)** Only then, could I start the real work on this book. Even though, two years is the time-frame the neurologists put on any improvements, this instance should encourage you to never give up hope. I can not tell you, what a big difference this made for me! So you see, the best may be yet to come. (Being a Cockeyed Optimist can't be all bad.)

Many are worse off than I. I am not writing this to complain. I know I am lucky: Lucky to be alive. Lucky to have my sight. Lucky to have partial memory… the memories I had possessed before the SHOCK. I had always read a lot and was aware of the World about us. I remember the Korean and Vietnam wars, and various skirmishes; invasions of Grenada and Panama. But, I also remember the Cold War ended with the Fall of the Berlin Wall, and there was a Mid-East Peace Accord. With our enlarged World, there were a lot of "people helping people" to live a better life. The World has changed a lot since my Crisis: There was something in Haiti and Bosnia. And starvation in Somalia. There was something about a Presidential Preference and then a Presidential Selection. During these *National Crisis's*, we couldn't even get International News! Let's not forget Desert Storm. (Okay, so I did forget. Just, don't ask for dates or details. There will always be one exception: 9/ll. Even I, can never forget this! I just equated the 911 Emergency number, with the biggest emergency we've ever seen.) For one who had always kept up with the latest news of the world, it was quite a blow… not being able to read and comprehend news, nor, retain the information. I found the TV News, with its stories and pictures, was easier for me to comprehend. I'm left without newspapers, books and magazines. Oh, I can enjoy them for the day... just won't remember what I've read tomorrow. (Anything worth remembering, has to be clipped and put in a file for future reference.) I know you are thinking, this can't be all bad; we are taught to think on things that are ***of good report.*** I don't recognize many of these reports, that would qualify as "good." Certainly, The Fall of the Berlin Wall, and the Mid-East Peace Accord are two.

For some brain injury victims, repeated brainwashing, may be helpful in getting the news across, but most people can comprehend what is being said, the first time they hear it. Even this brain injured person can do that! Though it is slowly absorbed, it is absorbed; and, it is all mine, for the day.

Repeated pandering and propagation of useless information, was even more confusing for everyone; much less, the brain-injured person. Remember, for many of us, the news was looked on as something new; we had forgotten yesterday. Still, the "Preference" and "Selection" stories, should not be choice subjects for any repeating (or should we say, "competing"?) Newscast. They would be better served, for what they are; an on-going saga of some (hopefully) ***short-running*** Soap Opera. So, **GIVE US A BREAK!!**

I tell myself, "It is better to have no feeling than to have constant pain." Some are in pain 24 hours a day. GOD Bless them. May they find comfort.

The symptoms of those suffering from a Lightening Strike or the Electrical Current Burns are as varied as the victims themselves. Like my meat loaves, no two alike. What we all need is compassion and understanding without pity and condescension. I am thankful for the many who made the effort to understand. It makes my life so much easier.

I cry for the person who was lost,
but I'm learning to live with the person I've found.

SHOULD I CLEAN IT UP ?!

I would guess that I could white-wash this paper,
but that might take away from the caper.

Sure, I could re-write this book,
taking some people off-the-hook.

I suppose I could wash this paper white;
making everyone into a Royal Knight.

But, what good would this do,
if the colors were not true?

I could take-back things, I wouldn't say.
What good would that do, anyway?

Words that are *Written-On-The-Wind*,
Will never be taken back again.

Denying the things that will be;
would that set my journey free?

Wishing people to be what they're not,
can not cleans the dirty spots.

What's right for them may not be,
the things that I would choose, for me.

We can not judge our fellow man,
So I've come back to where I am.

Leaving all of the these faults in the past,
returning to something I can grasp.

To see the best in everyone;
A philosophy, that is seldom wrong.

CHAPTER 11

THOSE FIVE STAGES OF GRIEF.

THOSE FIVE STAGES OF GRIEF.....

Everyone has heard about them, but never think of them when referring to ourselves. After all, we are strong. We are mature. We can handle anything that comes our way.

1. **Denial**? I know it happened. I have always looked reality in the face. No illusions. What has happened, happened. You can't change the past. Water under the bridge, etc. I am too intelligent to deny any of this. **(SURE!!)** I will dedicate myself into getting back to the way I was; no matter how long or how difficult, it might be. BUT, I've denied so many aspects of this SHOCK, I don't know where to begin. From day one, it was, "I will be alright tomorrow."....but tomorrow never came through, for me. "Just wait until the burning stops; then things will clear up." Never happened! "If I could just get rid of the FOG, I will think sharply and clearly again." "I just need to be patient and wait." (The slow motion persisted.) I will go on with some part of denial, for the rest of my life. When I have a really bad day; a day when my problems are so obvious to the rest of the world, I am crushed. It certainly should not be a big surprise to me, after all of these years. I want to be perceived as normal so badly, I kid myself into believing that I am. When I have a day of the "loss for words" in every sentence, I am tempted to say nothing. Try that! It doesn't work. You would just have to explain the, "Is something wrong?" A matter of symptoms perpetrating other symptoms. Just more problems to deal with. (Note, I never called them disabilities; I was so sure that this was all, *just a temporary condition.*)

2. **Anger**? I suppose I have anger about touching that faulty elevator button.... after all, many had received

little jolts before me; and many will have received jolts after me. I have most anger toward the hospital for allowing a possible life-threatening situation to persist for so many months. These are elevators used by the public, as well as patients and employees. I even found myself wishing others might know how I felt... you know, just a little jolt leading to my set of symptoms, for just an hour or two... maybe a day. <u>Then, they would understand</u> this tragedy! (But, reason would tell us, the extent of my injuries could never be a temporary thing. I've lived that denial.) The anger was heightened by the Hospitals attempt at minimizing the seriousness of the SHOCK, while degrading my integrity. Clearly, they have no conscious! (Perhaps, just very stupid!)

3. **Bargaining**? Sure, I see it now. I have always been that "Cock-eyed Optimist." I kept thinking that everything would be better tomorrow. When that didn't happen, I'd think "next week," "next month," or "next year." All the time, whining to my neurologist, "Can't I try some sort of speech therapy to help me remember words, help me learn to read and retain information, make my reactions and reflexes quicker???" (Of course, it all seems so silly now; but THEN, I was serious.) God Bless the patience of the Neurologist!! She would simply say that, "Only time will bring improvement; if indeed, there was to be any. You are very fortunate to have your memory of the past; some are left with no memory. There is ATTENTION DEFICIT with short-term memory, so therapy would not help. It could take nine months (then, eighteen months; then, 2-3 years; etc.) of slow and steady improvement, to reach your permanent degree of ability." **I didn't want to hear that!** Surely, something could be done! I'm in the medical field, for crying out loud! (And that is exactly what I was doing, *CRYING, OUT LOUD*.) As a nurse, I knew that repetition was <u>the way</u> to improvement for some stroke patients. I would, at least, try! I had started

right away, working with my slow hand. I found that my typing had many of the letters juxtaposed. It was not difficult to figure out what was happening... one hand was slower than the other.... letters normally hit by the right hand, came in slower. (They still do.) What was difficult to understand, was the reason for the slow hand.... it was not physical, but a neurological defect. Somehow, in a constant *FOG*, with Short Term Memory and Attention Deficit, this fact was not getting through. I needed to feel that I could do something to help my condition; even though, many of my symptoms would be permanent. I would work tirelessly, with the mouse of my husbands computer, playing Solitaire. Hey, don't knock it, it worked. (Psychologically). The typing mistakes seemed fewer. (Or, I should say, my corrections became faster and less irritating.) I could even sit down at the computer and determine how sharp I would be for the day. If I could play Solitaire without glitches, I could write a letter, shopping list, clean a drawer, etc. Yet, no amount of bargaining would cure the typing errors. This is a neurological problem; the hand/brain coordination is flawed. The slow hand is permanent. I had kept telling myself, "If I just work hard enough, long enough, I will overcome these problems." Little did I know, my *Bargaining Chips* had run-out long ago! I would find other ways of dealing with my "Problems." TIME is plentiful, now.

4. **Depression**? Now, what normal person would ever become depressed over a fact of life? What's normal? I found out real quick. After four years, the Neurologist told me that I had had all of the improvement that I could expect. I should accept my limitations and get on with my life. **I cried!** I had needed a good cry, for a long time. "The can-do girl" suddenly couldn't! But wait! What does she know? No one can be sure? It's been four years, but that doesn't mean I'll stop trying. I could hardly see to drive home, I was crying so. This was truly

a low-point for me. The lowest point in my entire life! (God works in mysterious ways…) I turned on my radio and the song "Hero" was playing. It was the boost I needed. Of course, I'll be strong enough for this, too! I snapped to my senses and never looked back.

5. **Acceptance**? I had always avoided harsh, degrading words when referring to my condition. I guess I was pretending I was not really that bad! Instead I used "twenty-minute delay," "It takes time to assimilate information," "reaction time is delayed," "Everything is in slow-motion," "I have a retarded response," etc. It wasn't until my evaluation by a Psychologist that I realized I had avoided the reality of my condition…I had denied it by using <u>anything but</u> the accepted words. Depression had become *MELANCHOLY.* As I spoke aloud to the therapist, I found myself saying things I would never have considered before. After listing the symptoms and residual affects of my condition, I said, "I guess, what it all boils-down-to is this, I am *SLOW* mentally and have a *RETARDED* response." (I would guess, that my acceptance of my condition is complete. It certainly took long enough!) Of course, I resent the outcome!! This was a horrible accident, that need not have happened! We hope others will learn from my experience. It can happen to anyone. From this day forth: **This will <u>not</u> be <u>a *disability*</u>, but <u>a *CHALLENGE.*</u>**

This was the day that defined what was left of "ME." I had come through a terrible ordeal, true. Now, I would have to get on with my life, accepting my limits; facing the challenges. When I think of all of the time I wasted, struggling to prove to everyone I was going to overcome these challenges and return to *Normal* again, I realized how tired it made me. It was all physically and mentally draining. It consumed me. I was constantly looking for new ways of fighting this reality, when I really **wanted to prove to myself** that *This Can-do Kid Rides Again!* It took years to convince myself that some things cannot change; and, that is alright.

I learned to laugh again, by laughing at my-self. I wish I could say that I learned to sing again. (Well, I did; but only remember the words of songs I had sang before touching the elevator button.) There are great new songs, but I must simply listen to enjoy. I won't retain the words. Let's face it, the excitement of a beautiful song, is always a joy. Many will claim that singing is an effective coping mechanism. Now, scientists are telling us that people who sing, increase their longevity. I can see that. You can always find a song to fit your mood. Like poetry, a song is soothing to the soul. Nothing ever seems so bad, too difficult a challenge, nor any situation impossible, with a song. Do you think that it is because someone else *has been there* with you? The person who wrote the song, probably experienced the situation they wrote about. Everyone who chooses, carries a song in their heart. They may not sing out-loud; but quietly, to themselves. You may hear some humming, or whistling. For my husband, when you hear him whistling "The Impossible Dream," you know he is having trouble getting that oil filter off of the car, or traffic is delaying his progress. (For him, it is "The Impossible Dream;" for me, it is "One Moment in Time.") Whatever the circumstances, *Music Makes It Magic.* I will live again, with a song in my heart. I have recaptured that ***piece of solace***. The world is a beautiful place.

Sure, I miss the old "ME." I still reminisce about the person and the *personality* of the past. I'm working hard at recreating that old personality, that was the REAL ME; I'm coming along. That "OTHER PERSON" is dealing with the disabilities. Fortunately, I don't remember much about the present "ME," and that is just as well. When I read back over my diary, I'm still a bit embarrassed. Let me say to "ME" and the rest of the world, **"Get over it!"** I may say the wrong words, have a loss for words, or even utter an occasional cuss word; **but,** just as I know that the "lawnmowers" are really windmills, **I do know, who I really am,** also. I am that lady of integrity and grace! Through it all, there was never a doubt. In whatever condition, I am once again, pleased to be me. **(A legacy is not determined by ones disabilities, but by what is accomplished despite the disabilities.)**

* * * * * * *

As it came to me that I should write about this experience, I wondered "HOW?!" I had seen an interview with former President Carter, in which he said that GOD always answers prayers: Sometimes, HE says "YES," sometimes, HE says "NO," and sometimes, HE says "You've got to be kidding!" I'm walking in a FOG, everything is in slow-motion, I can't remember material, I'm disorganized, my right hand is slow, I can't research anything.... why, **it could takes years!** (For one brief moment, **I was telling God,** "You've got to be kidding!") I'm ashamed, as I drag a few thoughts from my heart: I can do all things.... **(No time limit.)** HIS grace is sufficient.... **(We'll find the way to do it.)** If I persist; forgetting those things which are behind, and reaching forth to the things that will be.... **(We'll make it happen!)**

I DO SEEM TO HAVE THE PICTURE OF MY NEAR-ELECTROCUTION BURNED ON MY MIND.

* * * * * * *

CHAPTER 12

RECYCLED

RECYCLED……

Just as we shred our office papers, gather glass bottles into one container, aluminum cans into another, and newspapers, yet into another; re-cycling becomes a way of life. The products are chopped, ground, or melted and formed into products of renewed use. We feel we are doing something that can make a difference in our environment. It feels good and righteous. So too, we learn to recycle life's experiences. They are considered, sorted, evaluated, retained or tossed out with the rest of the garbage. So it goes…

As it had come to me that I should write about this experience, I had not wanted this job. I had not wanted to dredge-up past hurts and disabilities. We optimist avoid negativity, and cling to a positive out-look. You look for a way of making negativity, positive. How can we help others going through the same thing? Write about it, so everyone will know what we are going through. Perhaps the one thing I was trying to ignore, was the fact that I needed to recapture that *essence* of the person I used to be. When we think we have over-come the past, it often raises its ugly head. While taking a college course on *Neonatal ALS*, the instructor started the class by reminding us of the large number of women who have miscarriages; then, asked how many of us had miscarried and how many times. There were a few of us, but I had the distinction of having had the most miscarriages, so I became the unwilling spokesperson. Thinking that I had successfully put that part of my life behind me, I was surprised to find myself in tears. All of the well-meaning people had done more damage than they could have ever imagined. Twenty-five years later, I was sitting in a class, weeping for my loss. So the advise of "Keeping a stiff upper lip," "You're young. You can always try again," and "It's natures way of getting rid of an imperfect pregnancy," had not eased the *psychological miscarriage*. You are given that Mothering Instinct to protect and care for the young.... that doesn't go away. Perhaps, I really needed to write this book for *CLOSURE*, more than anything else. I guarantee, there is nothing left unsaid about this *miscarriage* (of justice). There will be no surprises, in my future. (Short Term Memory can't be <u>all</u> bad.) I can finally get on with my life. I had always been happy with the *person* I was. This book taught me to be happy with the person, I had become; looking forward to the person, I will be. I am even gathering-up some of *my old self*, by writing this book. Thanks, I needed that!

Everything progressed so slowly; but, it did progress! Time was passing me by, but I wouldn't remember it. I needed constant reminders of any progress. As I struggled on, writing the book, I found my "up-bringing" interfering. My Grandmother was the epitome of a "Women's Libber." She taught us to be strong: Girls were every bit as strong as boys and could do anything they could do (and probably better.) We could accomplish anything, if we just set our minds to it. I have always been that "Can-Do Girl." That determination is a part of my essence that will never change. I'm sure my Grandmother would be proud. While, I've always been my own person, I've had that desire to make my world a better place. We were taught that, if we were miserable, that was no reason to make others miserable. With this in mind, I felt the need to make my readers comfortable, even if this was an uncomfortable subject. Not so much of a "Disease to Please," as it was a try for "Humorous Relief." Aside from the Attention Deficit Episodes, I would find myself weaving bits of my BC life (before the crisis) into the manuscript, to soften this tragedy. I hope it doesn't take away from the seriousness of the subject. Sometimes, it is necessary to visit your past, in order to see where you've been and marvel at how far you've come, to realize the possibilities of what you are capable of achieving, still. So, this is it! **Suddenly, I understood**.

This is **what my History Teacher had been trying to tell me.** We are never too old to learn!

For those who thought that I had fallen off of the face of the Earth, after walking away from the ER that day; I apologize. Some people were like a small child picking a scab, the wound can never heal; and, may in fact, destroy you. The less-astute will see you as defective and a reject to society; looking to harass and belittle your progress, while taking advantage of your situation. Though you know you are not that reject, do you really need *"scab-pickers"* following you around? Addicts face the same truth: There will come times, you will have to set yourself free of the past, in order to get on with the future.

In reality, I should never have been put under the pressure of a work schedule. Can you imagine pushing-on through that FOG, trying to make sense of what was being said in slow-motion; and struggling to decipher doctors' orders (when you know it is difficult enough to read their writing), having difficulty finding the next line of print, without repeating the same line. As I labor to write this book, I see that I should have been given a **Medal for Bravery**, under extreme duress. And the novelty of it all is, I survived the test of my mettle. No, I realize now, I should not have been working; but, that was then. I should have been on Workers' Compensation. Still, the constant problems I encountered, kept me using that defective brain, and left me little time to worry about my condition; only striving to *overcome* my condition… As if I could. I would only learn to *cope with* conditions I could not control. Now I wonder, "Where was my Patient Advocate?" But again, I realized most had not recognized the extent of my injuries. This was all, one **losing battle**, from the beginning; ***or, was it*** the experiences I needed, in order to write this book?

Most experiences are good and we treasure them in our hearts. Sometimes, people betray you. You don't allow *negativity* to linger. Put it behind you. I have a saying: "Your heart is only so big. If you fill it with hate, you won't have room for love." We learn from all experiences, good or bad. They are always lessons we need to know. What you do with them is up to you. Most of us, put the bad ones behind us and get on with our lives. Negativity, begets negativity. A Positive Person Possesses Pure Pleasure in living each day to the fullest. We have seen the bumper stickers asking, "Have you hugged your kid today?" A good message. I think we need one that says, "Have you had a good laugh today?" Life is too short to miss one beautiful thought, one beautiful sunset, one beautiful face, or miss one beautiful song. **RECYCLING COMPLETED!** You have made your environment a better place in which to live.

CHAPTER 13

WHAT REALLY HAPPENED?

WHAT REALLY HAPPENED??

I WISH I KNEW !! I'm still standing on the outside, looking in; removed from the sorrow of this changed life. I stand afar, looking at this pitiful person, trying to assess her situation; yet, helpless to change her prognosis. It's as if this were happening to someone else. Suddenly, I step back into this reality and say, "Hey, that's me! I don't want it to be, but it's me." "Now what?" And, I don't have the answer. (Or at least, the answer I'm looking for: *It was all a bad dream, but now it's over.*)

We are a curious people; nurses, especially. We want to know what makes people tick. We analyze every tragedy and wonder how it might have been prevented. What can we do with the results of the aftermath. How can we help this person? My Medical Log is my only connection to my progress, but it should help the medical field comprehend details, they could only imagine. I'm thankful for the many friends who realized I could not comprehend long, detailed explanations of anything; and so, whenever they found information on the subject, that was "short and sweet," they would send it to me. After all of this time and explanations, it still comes down to the same old conclusions: ...The Electrical Trauma caused multiple injuries; many of which will last a lifetime. Some stabilized, a few would improve, and some would get worse; many, may be yet to come. My Internal Medicine Doctor wonders about seizures, cancers, arthritis, etc., years down the road. I'm not looking for any more trouble than I already have.

Most doctors don't know what to make of electrical injuries. Where do they begin? How do they determine nerve damage? There are no tests that will show the extent of the damage to the nervous system. (Though, I have heard of a new procedure called neurography.) The tiny little damaged nerves have no voice; no advocate for treatment.

Still, precautionary diagnostic blood tests, EKG, and uninalysis would be a good start. This is usually routine for any trauma patient seen in the ER. How about x-rays of bone pain? Also, another "routine." There should be **baseline tests,** in the least, to watch for changes. This would be **a prudent start**. But, does this go far enough?

As I would read about other Electrical Injuries, I would find victims with similar symptoms. So why isn't there a comprehensive book on the results of these injuries? Perhaps, we victims haven't the ability to understand what is happening or explain what we are feeling. We can only try. OSHA'S report for 1992 showed 347 deaths due to electrocution in the workplace, but how many more survive with these life-altering injuries? (And, how many occur in the garage or kitchen of the private home?! How many go uncounted, as mine did?) I suspect that the reason we are not talking about the subject, is because it is like seeing a ghost… No one would understand, so keep quiet. Most people are scared of things they do not understand, but if there are so many of these injuries with long-lasting effects, it's time to admit they exist, and do a study on them. (Over 5 million Americans are living with disabilities caused by Traumatic Brain Injuries.) While it is true that every victim may have a separate set of symptoms, we should stress all variables possible. I can only speak of my trauma. Maybe the World was waiting for the Nurse, with the first-hand experience, to explain her plight. Let's educate and help prevent this life-altering sentence for others. It's the least we can do for victims, who cannot do for themselves. And, it's the least we can do to help prevent others from falling victim. As I draw this book to a close, there have been two more construction injuries, involving electrocution; just in my county alone, in the past three months! Would my book have prevented these accidents? Probably not, but it would give the information needed, to handle the First Aid. (If only there were as much interest in this phenomena as there is in UFOs and Angels.)

As the daughter of an electrician, it's easy for me to understand electrical current doing so much damage. (And, if you grew up with a family of auto mechanics, you would know all about cars, by the osmosis of being around them.) As water seeks its own, electricity rides the currents of fluid. Sure, we laughed at the old murder mysteries, where the villain throws a radio into the bathtub or a hairdryer into the hot-tub, *to do someone in.* Not as far fetched as you might think. Why do you think there are warning labels on all electrical appliances? You could be electrocuted! Water is a great conductor of electricity. But, this would not be the old bathtub filled with water, as a volume conductor; but rather, the body itself has become an internal volume conductor. Think of the fluid within and how much water is contained in the body; no escaping that. All the blood, tissues, reservoirs and tiny nerve pathways are conductive. (Yes, I was made aware of how conducive a full urinary bladder could be.) Current will follow the path of least resistance; hitting the oxygen-rich arterial blood of the heart, pumping it straight to the brain via an express transport of a millisecond.

I wish I had been able to refresh my knowledge base and research the latest advances for the Electrical Burns. (Though, advances have been few.) This ability would have made my plight easier. Still, research and retaining information remained beyond my neurological abilities. When the FOG lifted, the uninterrupted Attention Deficit is a little easier to work with. (Is that an oxymoron? Attention Deficit is a problem with interruption of thought.) Since the information I will read today, is gone tomorrow; I started outlining and highlighting the information in my diary and medical progress notes. It is easier to find, even if it is still beyond retention. I will draw on this store and knowledge gleaned from all of these years of Nursing (plus, the

Electricians Daughter) for explanations of the cause and effect, and some symptoms and treatments to be expected. OSHA government websites were a big help, also.

Have I said how grateful I am to have my memories of the past? Those years before I touched the elevator button? The past day doesn't come into play, anyway. My diary takes care of the information after the SHOCK.

We can only hope that Emergency Room Personnel would learn enough about electrical injuries, to treat the patient appropriately. (Sure, we all glossed-over the subject in Medical School or Nursing School; but most burns are contact burns, caused by house fires and auto crashes, etc. More emphases would be placed on these subjects. Perhaps, a refresher course is due.) No matter what the source of their current, all victims will have the current pass through their brains. OSHA website tells us that **True Electrical Current Burns are one of the most serious injuries you could receive and should be given immediate medical attention!**

So, do you still think that a "routine exam" might be good enough for this type of injury? This has been a Traumatic Brain Injury and a thorough Neurologic Exam is a MUST! We might see things differently, once we've read the facts.

* * * * * * *

As a refresher, all of we Emergency Room Personnel should have a basic understanding and the knowledge of **HOW ELECTRICITY WORKS:** Think of it like this: Operating a light switch is like turning on a water faucet. Behind the faucet or light switch, must be a source of water or electricity, with something to transport it, and pressure enough to make it flow. <u>With water</u>, the source is a reservoir or pumping station; the transportation is through pipes; and the force to make it flow is pressure, provided by a pump. For electricity, the source is the power generating station; current travels through electric conductors in the form of wires; and pressure (measured in volts), is provided by a generator.

* * * * * * *

ELECTRICAL CURRENT BURNS:

The most common shock-related injuries are burns. An electrical accident can result in an Electrical Current Burn, Thermal Contact Burn, Arc Burn, or a combination of burns.

Three types of burns can occur, when electric current contacts the skin:

Thermal Surface Burns happen when the skin comes in contact with hot surfaces of overheated electric conductors, conduits or other energized equipment. Heat and flames that accompany electric current, can cause clothing to catch fire, also. These burns usually destroy the surface skin and subcutaneous tissue underneath; which is bad enough, if it happens to you.

Arc (or **Flash Burns**) from current that ***does not*** pass through the body, but are the result of high temperatures near the body, and are produced by an electric arc or explosion. If high current is involved, these arcs can cause injury or start a fire. Extremely high energy arcs can damage equipment, causing fragmented metal to fly in all directions. Even low energy arcs can cause violent explosions in atmospheres that contain flammable gases, vapors or combustible dusts.

True Electrical Burns happen when the current ***does*** pass through the body. In these burns, the body has become a part of the circuit. And, a true electrical current injury is really more like a crush injury because it goes deep and often destroys muscle tissue and affects internal organs. Tissue damage is caused by the heat generated as the current flows through the body. **It is one of the most serious injuries you can receive and should be given immediate attention.**

Electricity travels in closed circuits. Its normal route is through a conductor. An **Electrical Shock** occurs when the body becomes a part of that circuit. The **severity of the shock** will depend on the amount of current flowing through the body (amperes), the path of the current through the body, and the length of time the body is in the circuit. Other factors include: the frequency (Alternating or Direct), the phase of the hearts cycle (meaning, even minimal shocks can cause cardiac arrest… i.e., even stun guns.), and the general health of the individual (young healthy individuals should have extended CPR… up to four hours.) The **effects of the shock** will depend on the type of circuit, its voltage, resistance, current, pathway through the body, and the length of time the body is in contact. The higher the voltage and amperage and the lower the tissue resistance, the greater the damage. Therefore, we say the severity of the injuries depends on the type and intensity of the current, the duration of the currents contact with the tissue, and the resistance of the tissue the current passes through.

We might be complacent and put this in a neat little box, surmising a high-voltage lightening strike with it's 12,000 - 200,000 amperage of direct current (DC) would cause more damage to the body. However, that low-voltage alternating current burn (AC), with little resistance, may produce the same amperage, and thus similar damage. Were you surprised to learn that a low-voltage AC shock can equal the damage of a high-voltage lightening strike? Why? The answer is quite simple: the amount of time spent in contact.

Lightening is usually of very brief duration; one-hundredth to one-thousandth of a second. OSHA warns us again: **LOW VOLTAGE DOES NOT IMPLY LOW HAZARD!** A **severe SHOCK** may cause a person to suffer internal hemorrhages and destruction of tissues, nerves, and muscles.

So you see, Shocks can be anything from a "buzz" to cardiac arrest; and the difference between the two is less than 100 milliamperes!

Simply put: whether the direct current of a Lightening Strike or the indirect current of a low-voltage Electrical Hit, the injuries can be the same. And, they can be massive! Most of them, will be hiding underneath that "*normal looking facade*." Unlike other burns, the True Electrical Current Burn may have unseen damage deeper in the muscles and organs, far from the point of any obvious peripheral injury.

As we cover **Effects** and **Severity** of a Shock, we need to focus on the two types of current that may be encountered and their characteristics:

Alternating current (AC) produces tetanic muscular contractions which can "freeze" the victims' hand to the circuit, resulting in prolonged exposure, which increases the damage. Instead of getting one shock, they are getting repeated shocks; over and over again! Herein lies the horror of alternating current. However, if the extensor muscles are excited by the electric shock, the person may be thrown away from the circuit; much like the convulsion of DC current.

Direct current (DC) tends to cause convulsive contractions, forcing the victim away from the exposure. Either type of these Current Burns can affect the body, by altering physiologic functions; like involuntary muscular contractions and seizures, ventricular fibrillation, respiratory arrest, etc. They can also produce thermal electrochemical damage, as the current radiates heat along its path. It may cause necrosis of the muscles and other tissues as the heat coagulates blood, clotting the vessels or causing rupture of red blood cells. Dehydration is found in every burn, but more so with True Electrical Burns. Vertebral and other skeletal fractures, along with muscle and tendon avulsion is possible. Hyperkalemia may be to a point, it affects the hearts function.

So then, with either type, you could expect a combination of any of the above.

Entrance and Exit Wounds: Electrical Current injuries can be puzzling, to say the least; but, they usually produce obvious entrance and exit wounds; and, some not so obvious! You will have to check closely. They may be very small and painless; or, they could be quite large and explosive-looking, with a great deal of pain. These wounds may give you an idea of the extent of the burns and their pathway; however, the size will not indicate the severity. Blisters may form, when water vaporizes from the tissues. (Mine was **"spatter" burns** on both hands and arms, **and** the hole **burned** in the mucous membrane of the right **nasal septum**, exposing the cartilage.)

Another effect that will be paramount, is the ***Pathway*** taken **through the body**: Head and Thorax (between the base of the neck and the diaphragm) are more likely to cause immediate death, due to the involvement of the cerebral respiratory center or heart. Hand to Hand (horizontal) crossing the chest, is more likely to cause ventricular fibrillation than the Hand to Foot. Oh yeah? And where does that leave me? Darn lucky to be alive, I guess. My current had traveled two paths, at least. I had received ***Hand to Hand*** AND ***Head to Toe!*** I thought I had some real news for the rest of the World about this; but my doctors were quick to point out the fact that all three types of shocks could occur at once, as well as many different pathways taken.

We refer to our nerve pathways as the body's *electrical system.* Guess what? My *electrical system* has just been short-circuited, over-loaded and fried! No matter where the electricity enters your body, it is going to circulate through your brain. The type and duration of the current, will determine the extent of damage. The injuries are caused by the transformation of electric energy into heat. It stands to reason, when you think of it: As electric energy forms heat, the exterior burns will cool more quickly, while the deeper tissue will continue to radiate more heat. **Even the linings of my body cavities were burned.**

One study equated electrical injury to that of irradiation. I could see that. Even my entrance and exit wounds became more evident, the first few days; the "spatter burns" on my arms and wrists were reddened and had various stages of healing water blisters, while the hole in the membrane of my right nostril became larger, whiter and more obvious, as time progressed. It seems the burning became worse instead of better, the first month or two. (You will need to think of this patient as just a different type of **Burn Patient.)** What can be so devastating, is the fact that you can look so normal on the outside; inside, the burning continues.

You see, with alternating current, you are being shocked, repeatedly; and it seems to me, the constant reversing of polarity, might cause you to "*cook*," as you would in a microwave. (Or, at least, that's how it seemed to me. I felt "well-done." I felt like a piece of meat being seared on the outside, then placed in the oven, to slow-cook the insides.) That may have been a bit graphic, so let's go back to *cooked*, or, *browned* and *roasted.* **Low-frequency AC currents are usually three to five times more dangerous than DC currents** of the same voltage and amperage. **And**, AC current, is **more likely to cause death**, also. (A surprising fact, the *Electricians' Daughter* really hadn't thought about. We were taught to be careful around all electricity; because it can kill!) In general, whether a DC or AC Shock, the higher the voltage and amperage, = the greater the damage: i.e. A defective household lamp, as opposed to a powerful defective **HOSPITAL ELEVATOR!!!**

Because the current will flow through the brain, every lobe is vulnerable, and we will all have some brain involvement; every one of us, to differing degrees. We have just received a **Traumatic Brain Injury!** No matter what the source of our current, we share many of the same symptoms. As to what the future holds? Whatever happens, happens. You deal with it.

As a nurse, having taken care of these **Burn Patients** before, I understood the seriousness of these types of Electrical Current Burns. A severe Shock, (as I had received), can cause considerably more damage to the body than is visible. Yet, at present, many patients are simply abandoned, due to the unknown. I suppose, worse yet, is the tendency to prescribe mind-altering drugs. They may receive narcotic pain medication for relief of their excruciating pain; or a tranquilizer for the hysterical *head cases* (by which, many will be defamed.) The brain has enough change to contend with. We don't need to struggle with more confusion and delayed responses. You must always consider the possible internal damages. Not an easy task! There may be internal hemorrhages, destruction of tissues, organs, bones, nerves, and muscles.

I instinctively treated myself as a *burn victim*; while my ER Doctors were treating me as a *head case,* and I was in such a confused state, I could not fight for my rights to treatment. I just knew that there was something terribly wrong. For any treatment, it was obvious, I would be on-my-own. (Please, don't consider **the inability to form**

sentences, a sign of fright; it **is a neurological problem!** But, of course, you should know that!)

I was careful to get enough liquids. Every "*Burn*" patient will have some degree of dehydration, no matter how mild the Shock was thought to be. I could feel the extent of my many burns and knew I would need to flush away the residual toxins of the damaged cells and would require a balanced diet with added Calories and Vitamin C, for tissue repair. In my state of confusion, any other therapies, were beyond my grasp. No other medical help or treatment was forthcoming; I had been discharged three hours after the fact, to drive myself home; I was on-my-own! (Maybe that's a good thing! The doctors didn't seem to know what was going on.) After a while, you realize it may all be just a part of a gigantic ***Cover-Up.*** No one can be that dumb!

We know that all burns cause dehydration, but I didn't need a reminder; I could feel my burns, day and night. I had no one to keep track of my daily progress. Here's the glitch: I should have been monitored for fluid replacement. In this type of burn, you cannot use the standard Burn Charts for fluid replacement. Dehydration is worse in the True Electrical Burn. I suppose it is because, you can't really see the burns hiding beneath the surface. (While all fluid replacement is carefully monitored, we emphasize it here. Initially, muscle damage is from the currents direct effect; later it is from the disruption of the blood supply. These muscles have been injured and already have swelling; fluid over-load would further decrease vascular integrity, causing increased muscular congestion, perhaps, leading to gangrene and amputation.) How can you possibly ascertain the degree of internal burns? You can't! Their Intake & Output will be your indicator for fluid replacement. Try to keep the output between 70 and 100ml/hr. if indicated.

I had just received **one of the most serious injuries** a person could receive and should have been given immediate medical attention and observation. Instead, I had had, what we call "a drive through" or "peek-a-boo" examination. Some ER Doctors are unaware of the effects of Electrical Current Burns or the Emergency Care required. As the days trickled past, even in my state of confusion, it would become quite evident to me, the Hospital cared little about my wellbeing; but rather, the publics perception of this "*Great Community Institution of Compassion. Always here for you!*" **NOT !** I'm just a number; THEY seek bottom-line.

"Since the numbness in your hands disappeared, what's your problem?" I'm afraid, it would seem, some "*Doctors of the old school*" still consider the symptoms of women, less crucial than the symptoms of men. Always ready to give someone the benefit of the doubt, I figured the doctors were too busy to investigate something they couldn't see. Wait! They investigate unseen medical mysteries every day!

Taking advantage of my disabilities started early, didn't it? At the time of my slow assimilation, I did not see it. "The numbness of the hands disappeared, so, what's the problem?" "What's the problem?!" There are many! And many may be yet to come.

Neurological deficits may occur, if the Central Nervous System is affected by vascular disruption or demyelinization. This is why, on admission, a thorough Neurological Exam is a MUST! A return to function, after direct nerve damage is uncommon. Deficits of cerebral, cerebellar, spinal cord and peripheral nerve function may be evident immediately after the injury or may have a delayed onset. **Direct Nerve Damage** at the onset, leaves little hope of a return to function. (This is what I found so difficult to comprehend, in my days of the "FOG." I kept pushing against all hope, to "over-come" the obvious *damage.* As if I could! But, that "Can-Do Girl" kept trying.)

Generally speaking, immediate and early deficits involving nerves <u>not</u> directly damaged, will show spontaneous resolution, in time. But, the **Late Appearing Peripheral Nerve Deficits,** leave a <u>return to function unlikely</u>. Though these Delayed Neuro Syndromes can occur days, weeks, or many months after the initial electrical trauma; these **damages are permanent**. (I don't know why, but studies show that Motor Nerves seem more sensitive to current injury, than do Sensory Nerves.)

If there is injury to the spinal cord, there may be myelopathy; wasting of the muscle, due to nerve injury. Immediate symptoms of spinal cord injury are considered the result of direct neuronal insult and are more often transient than are those of later onset. Transient or permanent spinal cord lesions and motor deficits can occur from the disruption of the spinal cord's blood supply, also. Much like the Neuro deficits, the later onset of spinal injuries are more apt to be permanent.

Compression fractures of vertebral bodies can occur from the tetanic contractions of the paraspinous muscles. It can happen! My **Whiplash** would have been expected, when my head was violently thrust backwards (Hyperextension), from the jolt of the SHOCK. This can cause an intradural bleed, swelling and cord compression from a vertebral fracture or ruptured disk. But, when I complained of neck pain from my whiplash, it was considered the reaction of an excited lady or a try for a few days of paid compensation, by condescending doctors.

I was not able to tilt my head backwards or look up at the ceiling, for four years. When did that change? Why, when an X-ray tech forced my head back for an x-ray of the right shoulder injury, four years later; there was a definite *CRACK* sound. The forcing should never have been done, but, for better or worse, I've been able to use my neck since then. The forcing could have, just as easily, paralyzed me;

and should never have been done. Still, I lucked-out, this time. (I was curious about the size of my **spinal disc** after the SHOCK… they were half the thickness, as before; even though my bone density was like someone half my age.)

Vessels can be burned so badly, blood does not flow freely. Even small vessels of distant organs can be cauterized by the heat. This can lead to gangrene of extremities or infarcts of soft tissue in the organs. Many, *apparently superficial burns*, may be deceptive when very little happens for several weeks; while, sloughing is slowly occurring, over a wide area. One can see how the whole body is vulnerable. The subtle injuries, hidden in unsuspecting regions, make these patients the equivalent of an auto accident victim; likened to **Crush Injuries.** It will take constant vigilance of every system. As with any crush injury, Doctors will be ordering a plethora of tests, searching for the unknown. The victim should be followed, to rule-out delayed damage to extremities, muscles and all organs; while watching for kidney failure, liver impairment, abnormal blood sugar, gallbladder disease, a paralytic ileus, intestinal perforation or dysfunction **(Aperistalsis)** etc. Cataracts, seizures, and cancers may develop immediately or years later.

Sensory damage often occurs in front of the heart. **Nerves of the hearts vessels** can be affected. Mine was in the form of the **Syndrome-X Angina**. This is an impairment in normal endothelial function of the coronary microvasculature, causing inadequate coronary flow reserve, due to inappropriate vasoconstriction. In short: when one exercises, is stressed, or cold, the coronary arteries lack the ability to dilate in order to meet the increased blood demand. Instead, the coronary arteries constrict distally, causing a lack of perfusion and myocardial ischemia (heart muscle injury); resulting in chest pain, despite normal, non-stenosed coronary arteries. With the **numbness under the ribcage**, it's a guessing game; any pain is felt on the outside of the ribcage. I'm on a calcium channel blocker and low-dose aspirin, daily. And, I'm doing well.

The only liver problem is **high cholesterol,** for which I am taking pravastatin. The **Gallbladder** had to be removed, due to the pain on top of the chest and on the back. Areas of vessel injury can cause necrotic areas in soft tissues of the pancreas, lungs, gallbladder, etc. Knowing that Sensory Damage often occurs in front of the heart and without the ability to feel anything under the ribcage, the pain had to be treated as a probable cardiac problem. It took an ultrasound of the gallbladder to differentiate between the two. The other organs seem to be alright, at present. (Or, at least, so it seems. Who would know, until something happened?)

Yes, there have been problems with **blood sugar**; but, not diabetes! There have been times when I would feel faint from low blood sugar. A sip of soda or a piece of fruit or candy, would take away the light-headedness. Soon after, I would be uncontrollably sleepy. The longest episode lasted about six months, intermittently; yet, blood glucose remained normal.

I was beginning to think of mononucleosis, but no swollen glands. However, infarcts are common in soft tissues of the pancreas. I've learned that I must eat, when I first feel faint. No more of that ignoring lunch, while out shopping. (We girls are bad about that!)

Eye exams drive the doctors nuts. Occasionally, there will be a change for the worse, but by the time the glasses are made, my eyes have changed again. Sometimes, they are better than they've been in years. One ophthalmologist had suggested a test for diabetes. That test proved negative. (Perhaps, just the Rouge Roads, again.) You might think of this as a rather aggravating nuisance, but I am so thankful to have good sight, I'm willing to do anything to help maintain it. Due to allergies to drugs, I must use the Optomap (digital retinal imaging) to keep abreast of the health of my eyes.

I've had the expected **Cancer** and **Arthritis**. Now, **Cataracts** are a shadow on my horizon, also; though, I have no family history of cataracts. The predisposition to these, and many other problems, has been termed *a life-sentence*.

I was told some of the **motor/sensory problems** were from the current crossing the back of my spinal cord (some areas will be adversely affected, while others will not); but how could I blame one system, when everything is such a mysterious mess?

Burns from electricity can be so massive and wide spread; yet, invisible to the naked eye. As I've said before: My brain felt like a red, hot poker dwelt in the top of my head; and the occipital lobe, as if it were being soaked in a warm bath. A path of warmth crawled along the top of the frontal lobe, causing facial numbness. No one can fully understand what that *ever-present **FOG*** was like. It was a constant peripheral assault. It makes your "skin crawl." No, really! Every inch of my skin felt the soft wave of touch, but nothing was there.

You feel like something is brushing against you, from all directions at once. Everything is happening in slow motion. It's like, I never quite understood what was being said or what exactly I was observing. I think it was because of the delayed responses; or, were the delayed responses due to the inability to comprehend what was going on. After six years of the FOG, I found relief from that Hell, with daily does of Vitamin E. Somehow, the slowed responses seemed tolerable, without the FOG. I could spend the rest of my life, trying to figure out the slow motion… it is permanent. I have accepted that fact and will get on with my life. (How many forms of **APRAXIA** could you find?) How about the unbelievable pressure on the back of my head? It was not something that went away in a day or two (as I, and the ER Doctor, had hoped it might), but much of this pressure lingers today. These are **my** symptoms, but every victim will have their own set of symptoms, depending on the areas of damage.

With water being such a good conductor, there is no resistance. In my case, the floors had just been mopped, but there was no standing water visible; however, we could still feel the moisture in the air. The loud "clap" and "flash" with my experience, might have been brought on by the moisture. Even low-energy arcs can cause violent explosions. Be aware of your environmental surroundings; they count. Then again, I was touching a metal bed rail with the top of one hand, while it rested on top of the Monitor/Defibrillator, and had my metal writing pen in the hand that touched the elevator button. (And yes, metal is a great conductor of electricity, also.) If the extensor muscles are excited by the shock, the person may be thrown away from the circuit. I would guess, that is what saved me… the involuntary arching of my body and the arms flying up above my head. In that nano-second following the initial Hand to Hand surge, my eyes were open but I couldn't see; so, I ask :

WHAT REALLY HAPPENED?!

I had heard the loud CRACK; was aware of the heat in my arms, chest, brain, and thighs; the arms flying up and the body arched back farther than I thought a body could; my writing pen hitting the opposite wall behind me, with such force it ricocheted three times from wall to wall, back and forth across the hall; aware that I was falling forward, because my ankles would not hold me; reaching for anything to break-my-fall. Then, as my sight returned, I saw my pen, spinning on the floor, about two feet from my left hand. As I scooped it up, it was then, I realized what had taken place and that the heat at my

thighs had been incontinence of urine; my socks were soaked and my shoes sloshed. This can't be good! I'm stunned and in a daze. I feel like a two-year-old. I can't think clearly, and nothing is making sense. My brain had recorded it all, like a movie in slow-motion. In my movie, I feel no pain; until reality comes back again.

* * * * * * *

Since the involuntary action of incontinence was in that same nano-second, did the wet socks and shoes attract another path of current? (OSHA tells us blisters can; the current causes blisters which reduce the body's resistance and increases the current.) How about the metal pen to top of defibrillator path? Did that "fire" the defibrillator? So, was there really a double shock? Maybe a triple shock? Boy! Do I have questions! There are more mysteries than I can ever answer. For certain:

EVERYTHING STARTED WITH THAT FAULTY ELEVATOR!

Who would have thought that something that seemed so simple, could be so intense? We had never given Electrical Injuries much attention before. Now, we see how invasive it can be. Knowing it can involve any organ or system, means that a simple ***"Routine Exam"*** will not even come close to the amount of investigation it will take to discover all of the variables possible with this type of injury. Your work will be cut out for you! Not every victim will be a True Electrical Burn, but every Electrical Injury victim should be observed until the determination is made.

It is suggested, that every Electrical Injury victim be hospitalized for three day, in the least, after the Cardiac and Neuro statuses appear stable. They will be monitored and observed for adverse changes. (Doctors say that this is when Cardiac Arrest is most likely to occur. And, as the internal burning continues, so will the Neuro problems.) The Level of Consciousness may change suddenly and drastically.

After the Cardiac status, the Neuro state will be tantamount to all else. The Nervous System has been in contact with the current. Would you expect a stroke victim or other head injury patient to be alert and coherent? (Remember, all of us have had current circulate through our brains.) After having gone through this myself, I'm convinced that the patient with an electrical injury should also be treated the same way we treat one who has had a Heart Attack or a Stroke. In reality, we have suffered many small attacks, all over our bodies. Be alert for a failure in any of the systems. It can happen. All are vulnerable, after the burning of a **True Electrical Burn**.

No matter what, we know that these patients have had **Traumatic Brain Injuries**. This is why the Neurological Exam is so important. When you ask how they are feeling, can you really expect them to form logical thoughts, during an injury of this type? A big **NO. NOT LIKELY !**

Is it any wonder doctors would have problems assessing these victims? The internal burns make them the equivalent of the **Crush Injury** of an auto accident**.** You must constantly be searching for the unseen and the unknown. The best one can do, is to expect the unexpected. Every part of the body, is fair game. It has experienced a **Burning Trauma,** most of which may not be visibly apparent; and may get worse before it gets better... if ever. Perhaps we should treat them the same as a serious Motor Vehicle Accident. Any and all systems and organs can be involved. Therefore, we must monitor all. The main thing here, is for us to **Get Serious!**

For the Health Professionals: Your work is cut out for you! There may be Major Trauma, hiding under the façade of normalcy. You must consider the Total Person; now, and what lies in their future. The SHOCK is **not a one-time injury**. It can cause more damage than is visible; and, is often **only the beginning** in a **chain of events.** Involuntary muscle reactions can cause secondary injuries. We need to consider falls, cuts and bruises, internal hemorrhages, or explosive bone fractures; along with the destruction of tissues, nerves and muscles. Among other things, the Shock can easily lead to Renal Failure and Liver Disease. Lung and Intestinal infarcts or ileus can occur.

There is a wide variety of the <u>later effects</u> of the electrical burns and related injuries, leading to the delayed fatality or an extreme alteration of ones life. We might expect Cancers, Loss of Hearing, Cataracts, Blindness, Cholelithiasis, Diabetes, Loss of Memory or Loss of Abilities to perform everyday tasks that were once so easy, Amputations, AND worse yet, may be the Feeling of Worthlessness. You are not who, you used to be. So What? This was not your fault! See what you have to work with and accept the new you, with anticipation of the possibilities of tomorrow.

Many say the scary part is, there is no *statute of limitation* for us. No *time-frame* will set us free from our symptoms; just chance. Doctors who work with our problems, consider two years as the *normal* time-frame for any improvement. That is not set-in-stone. I have found little conquest, all along the way. Every burn victim has their own set of problems. Some will do well, while others will do poorly. Yet, we know there will never be a cure for every symptom. We stumble onto a cure, symptom by symptom. For some, the injuries caused by their Electrical Shock may well lead to delayed fatalities.

FIRST AID:

If you should come upon the scene of an accident you think might be an electrocution... **LOOK FIRST** at the surroundings. **DON'T TOUCH!** The person may still be in contact with the electrical source and touching them, may send the current through you. *** **IF HIGH-VOLTAGE** is involved, **STAND CLEAR!** (This means, at least, 60 feet away.) A live wire could bounce around and hit someone else. Contact building maintenance or the Power Company to turn off this power. ***

Yell for help and make use of that cell phone to **Call 911**. **For Low-Voltage:** If possible, **turn off the electricity,** by removing the fuse or pulling the main switch. If this is not possible, and you can see the low-voltage wire that is in contact with the victim, *You can move a low-voltage source away* from you and the victim. **Stand on a dry surface,** (such as a newspaper, blanket, or rubber mat, etc.); and **Use a non-conductive material,** (such as a dry broomstick, piece of plastic pipe, cardboard, fiberglass pole, pottery, glass, ceramic, etc.), to move the wire. You may also be able to pull the victim free from the wire with a dry piece of rope or towel looped around their arm or leg. Make every move with care, conscious of your surroundings, while helping the victim.

Once the victim is **clear of** the **electrical source,** check the person's breathing and pulse. If either is absent or very slow and shallow, initiate resuscitation immediately (**CPR**); continue, until help arrives. Since Electrical Shock victims fall into a special category for resuscitation, they will often need vigorous and prolonged CPR with fluid replacement, and yet survive. In some instances, the shock occurred while their own heart was in recovery (or rest cycle) and it caused cardiac arrest. Other causes are injury to the brains' control center, which controls vital organs, and of course, injury to the lungs/diaphragm or the heart directly. Although, these injuries may be complicated by internal hemorrhages and other internal injuries, with destruction of tissues, nerves, and muscles; yet, these victims stand a good chance of survival with prompt resuscitation and care. Though time is of the essence, **DO NOT PUT YOURSELF AT THE RISK OF SHOCK !** Move with care and remain calm and "centered" on the care you are providing.

If they are conscious but are pale or faint, lay the person down with the head a little lower than the trunk, and elevate the legs slightly. Be alert for deteriorating conditions, until the Ambulance arrives. Everyone receiving an Electrical Shock, must be hospitalized for treatment and observation, no matter how minor the shock was thought to be. A thorough Neurological Exam is crucial, on arrival; for accurate follow-ups. Keeping in mind, that underneath the facade of normalcy, may lie the devastation of a **True Electrical Burn**. The type of burn will determine the severity.

* * * * * * *

Just as there are differing degrees of Electrical Injuries, there may be differing degrees of **Lightening Strikes**: You may see arborescent tracings on the skin, (reminiscent of tree branches or spider webs), indicating the path. The effects of being hit directly by a Lightening Strike would be more severe than being stunned by a "close call" from a Bolt hitting a tree or other object nearby, or a swimming pool, etc.

In a pool, obviously, you would encounter drowning from stunned bathers. A fall, may lead to other injuries. Broken tree limbs can be another danger encountered. Always take note of the entire situation, before delivering care. Administer care as quickly as possible; but, don't put yourself in danger. You cannot solve a problem, if you become a part of it! All Lightening Strike Victims must be hospitalized for treatment and observation, no matter how mild the strike was thought to be, also.

For LIGHTENING STRIKES:

Storms seem worse and more frequent than before. I expected the usual storms, when we moved to the "Lightening Capital of the Country," but it was never this bad; however lightening storms are claiming more victims from all the states. Maybe Global Warming! Or perhaps, Global **Warn**ing? I don't know, but the storms seem bad.

We are seeing an increase in Lightening casualties. What can we do? Perhaps the best we can do, is avoid lightening.

The National Lightening Safety Institute tells us, when you see the thunderstorms forming, seek shelter in a strong building, away from windows and doors; turn off and unplug appliances, computers, power tools and televisions. Do not seek shelter beneath canopies, near trees or under small plastic shelters. Avoid water, high places, and open spaces. Avoid metal objects, such as fencing, machinery, motors or power tools. We're reminded that the first and the last strikes of the storm are most deadly. The last strike can be as long as 30 minutes after the storm has passed.

As the storm moves on, the first thing you can do for the Lightening Strike Victim, is check their Respirations and Pulse. (And NO, you cannot receive a shock from touching a lightening strike victim; however, be aware of the storm around you.) There is frequently Cardiopulmonary Arrest. It's vital to get circulation going as soon as possible. Statistics show that, up to two-thirds of the Lightening Strike

Victims survive, when given prompt treatment. With young, healthy individuals, CPR can take four hours; and they may still survive. CPR can be life-saving in such patients. Be aware that coma and neurologic deficits are common, immediately after injury, but may resolve in a few hours; yet some may last several days. (These patients should receive sustained artificial resuscitation in the hospital, as long as there is no evidence of brain death.) However, survival will still depend on the extent and severity of the injury.

When the Ambulance Arrives:

For you Everyday Heroes, who cared enough to learn CPR to make a difference and to help your fellow man, **WE THANK YOU!**

When the Ambulance arrives, they will assess the victim and take information from you rescuers as to what happened and what care has been given; (while continuing the CPR, if necessary.) The ABC's are always first priority!

The Emergency Medical Responders will have checked for an unobstructed airway; knowing that entrance and exit wounds can interfere with their breathing, if facial or neck wounds are present. Is their breathing adequate on its own? (There could be respiratory muscle paralysis and no respirations.) Their heart rhythm may be as mild as a little fast or a little slow, or as severe as Ventricular Fibrillation or Cardiac Arrest; all subject to rapid change. They will put the victim on Oxygen and a Cardiac Monitor, start IV's and insert a Urinary Catheter; working to stabilize the patient, before transport. They will have checked his Level of Consciousness (this is an on-going observation). Symptoms can be as mild as just feeling "weak" or as severe as seizures, and convulsions; subject to rapid change, also. While checking the ABC's (Airway, Breathing, and Circulation) are always first priority. Circulatory problems can be as mild as a high pulse and low blood pressure to burn shock (from fluid shifts.) From simple dehydration to burn shock, all will require fluid replacement. Since we cannot see the extent of the internal burns, we cannot determine accurate numbers for a Fluid Replacement Chart, we will have to depend on the patients urine output to keep abreast of fluid needs. Everyone must be vigilant for changes in any system, at any time. Why is everything subject to change? **As the electric energy transforms into heat, the damage continues.**

The Emergency Medical Personnel have placed the victim on a backboard, with a hard cervical collar, to immobilize and protect them from further injury. They are aware of the fact that the spine, along with ribs and long bones, can have fractures. Other musculoskeletal injuries could include dislocations, ruptured tendons, muscle contractures, and tremors. With spinal cord injury, any of these symptoms are possible, along with flaccid paralysis (wherein, the muscles are flabby, having defective or a complete loss of muscle tone.)

Pop Quiz: So, is this a Brain Trauma, a Burn Victim, a Crush Injury, or, possibly, a Stroke/ Heart Attack Patient???

Aware that all Electric Shock victims have had current pass through their brains, will automatically make this a **BRAIN TRAUMA** patient. Frequent Neuro Checks, a must.

As the electric current transforms into heat, it will go on radiating heat internally; therefore they are considered a **BURN PATIENT**.

As heat damages the vessels, it will impede blood flow to muscles, and cause infarcts to soft organ tissue. Injury to nerves can mean they will not be functioning properly and it will be up to the Professionals to be alert for changes; in any system, at any time. Much like an Auto Accident, we will consider this a **CRUSH INJURY**. Expect the unexpected.

If vascular disruption or demyelinization of the Central Nervous System occurs, watch for a multitude of problems. Even the nerves of the heart are affected. Since infarcts can occur most anywhere, watch the Level of Consciousness for decrease in ability to express themselves or understand what is happening, and their ability to move or feel sensation. Sorry, but they should be treated like one with an impending **STROKE** or **HEART ATTACK.**

(Correct answer: All of the Above, and more. Good Luck!)

AT THE HOSPITAL:

Chances are great, that CPR was initiated, in the field. The cardiac rhythm may have been reestablished and there is a patent airway with high-flow oxygen. The I.V. is going, for fluid replacement. An indwelling urinary catheter has been inserted to monitor the output. There was an ABG to assess for hypoxemia. A venous blood draw is done, for that plethora of tests. X-rays of the chest, spine and long-bones may have been done. An EKG was taken, and the patient had been placed on a cardiac monitor. You have stabilized the patient… or have you?! Keeping in mind, serious dysrhythmias may occur after the cardiac status appears stable, be ready to intervene appropriately; in case of Ventricular Fibrillation, Cardiac Arrest, or other possible lethal Arrhythmias.

Perhaps, the victim never lost consciousness. He may have arrived conscious, but dazed; a bit perplexed at the whole experience. There are few outward signs of trauma. You could consider him *lucky* and in stable condition; ready for discharge… or could you? Not so fast! On arrival, that thorough Neurological Exam is crucial; for evaluation and accurate follow-ups. The patient may have serious internal injuries, even if he has minimal external burns. And, if the Electrical Burn caused CNS injury, he may develop neurological complications, long after you consider him stable. Perform frequent neurological assessments. Be especially alert for Convulsions, Respiratory Depression and Respiratory Failure, also. As radiating burns may continue deep in the tissues, and can affect any system, one must be observant for changes in all systems.

If extremities are involved, keep elevated to prevent increased swelling from possible muscle injury. In which case, peripheral pulses will continue to rise the first 2 or 3 days. Contact the doctor, at the first sign of neurovascular compromise. With the impaired immune system, we watch for septic shock. If the injury is severe enough, amputation may be necessary. The sad thing is, this type of damage may not be apparent for 7-10 days after the injury. Careful observation, early on, may prevent severe consequences.

The first 24 hrs of rehydration must be followed closely. Watch carefully. Check output against symptoms and labs. All victims will have some degree of dehydration. For some, fluids by mouth may suffice, but most will be given fluids by IV. This allows for accurate measures of intake and output.

And, we all know that the urinary output will determine the amount of fluid intake needed. The patient must maintain the high caloric nutritional needs of a Burn Patient, also. Assess for the presence of bowel sounds, frequently; alert for ileus, perforation or other dysfunction. Weigh patient daily.

(With all of these observations and anticipated treatments, we can see why every Electrical Current Burn Victim should be hospitalized for three days, in the least.)

While every electrical injury may not be of a True Electrical Burn type, we need to observe the patient, until the determination is made. Both the Thermal Surface Burn type (which can cause clothing to catch fire), and the Flash Burn type, causes obvious burns to treat. You can see what you have to work on. But, remember, *ALL THREE TYPES CAN OCCUR AT ONCE*; and the most devastating will be the one which had the current surging through the body: **THE TRUE ELECTRICAL BURN.**

The Wake-up Call.

We seldom consider this *Marvelous Magic* known as electricity, which has become such a big part of our everyday life. Let's not let it take away any part of that life.

What can we do **to prevent these injuries**? I think we become complacent: Are you still using the hairdryer that you have to shake, in order to get it to work? How about that frayed electrical cord on the clippers? Plugging in the fan with the loose prongs? Leaving outlets uncovered, with a toddler in the house? Let's clean-up our act. What happened to "Safety, First?" We can replace or *do without* a piece of equipment, but we cannot replace or *do without* you or your toddler!

Companies, you <u>really</u> need to clean-up your act! Many seem aloof and uncaring. Why would you allow a dangerous situation to persist? Are you willing to gamble with the lives of your workers? Apparently so. We want to see more Company responsibility for the dangers in the workplace. Some companies do a good job. It's the others that give them all a bad name. If all companies tried to make a safe working environment, we wouldn't need OSHA. If the Company doesn't report the accident to OSHA, you should report it. If the family finds the patient incapable of reporting the incident, be an advocate, and report it to OSHA on their behalf. Unless there is a true accounting for these accidents, it will not be perceived a "real" problem. Like I say, not every person strives to live an honorable life.

We need to prevent these life-altering injuries. We must all be alert, for the things we can change. Accidents will still happen, when we encounter the unseen hazards. Though, in most case histories I've read, the victims were using defective electrical appliances or workplace equipment/machinery that had been giving hints of a defect; others had reported "buzzes," blown fuses, etc.; yet, the equipment was never checked or repaired. (Probably just *static electricity*! More like, "We don't want to spend the money," if the truth is known.) We can stop most of these types of accidents, but we have to step forward and demand change. **REFUSE TO USE** a tool or piece of equipment, if there is a question of its safety. It may be a *shock hazard.* You are too important to your family. Your friends and community need you. Let's all play-it safe.

If it blows a fuse, **REFUSE TO USE!**

* * * * * * *

OUT OF BODY.

I was out-of-body,
Looking back at me.
Thinking, "Really, I look so silly;
like some movie from a *slap-stick comedy*."

Aware of the pen ricocheting from wall to wall;
I'm lingering somewhere, here above it all.

I'm aware of what's happening, but feel no pain;
as if I'm playing a virtual video game.

Everything is a pinkish-tinged vastness;
like looking at my world through "*rose-colored glasses*."

(Wouldn't you know, even in this harrowing plight,
I would see things, in a positive light?)

"Look, my ankles are like jelly." They feel so weak;
as I crumble to the floor, in a useless heap.

My eyes are open, but I can't see.
Yet, I am afar, looking back at "Me."

Now, I am back with a *spinning pen*.
My eyes are open and I can see again.

THANK GOD!!!

I had felt the *tingling buzz* of the Shocks' hand-to-
hand path,
and am beginning to feel the Executioners' wrath.

Something is wrong, it doesn't compute!
I've been fitted into this prisoners suit.

In this suit, I am empty clear to the core.
I've never known anything like this before!

I have no rights, no choices to make.
It's all been decided by this terrible fate.

Suddenly, I'm like a good puppy;
"Whatever you say."
Boy! I had never been raised that way.

I'm caught in a FOG, all sounds seem to grow.
My hearing, assimilation, and responses are slow.

This state of confusion, you can't comprehend.
It goes on forever, without any end.

Where had it ended, the demarcation line;
between past memory, and present time?

At the precise moment, I could see my pen;
this was where my *altered life* began.

I could remember my past, just not the past day.
And, how could that happen, anyway?

Sure, I wish I could get <u>all</u> memory back again; but
Current Memories are archived by family and
friends.

They keep me laughing, so I'm having great fun.
By the stories they tell, there's fun for everyone!

So, if we've met, I hope I've *Made-Your-Day*;
I'm sure you've made mine. (I just won't
remember.)
So, what can I say?

THANKS!

(by Windy Wynn)

CHAPTER 14

LIFE GOES ON.

LIFE GOES ON...

Life goes on, with all of its sweet mysteries and mighty trying miseries. That's life! In these few years, I've had other distractions in my life. With the usual deaths, came the usual births. As Spring follows Winter, it is to be expected. Then the unusual joys of traveling to Florida for a nice wedding. (No, not one of our four children, but my 80-year-old father-in-law.) There were other weddings and a few divorces; promotions and job losses; the fit and the ill; the better-off and those who could be better-off. These are all the results of life. We have had great visits to and from friends and family. I've enjoyed great sight-seeing, biking, and hiking. There were the usual time-consuming distractions of work schedules and finances. Income Taxes, State Taxes, and User Taxes sure kept me on my toes, mathematically. (It seems that side of the brain is still functioning well. Though, that is not the side I would choose, let us be grateful for any ability.) We really are blessed. What a beautiful world!

I've accepted this condition, *BUT* It's the "Thumb-in-the-Eye" that hurts. That darn *Fogginess* hung-in-there for six long years. The *Slow Motion* and *Delayed Reaction Time* was a part of the problem I could learn to deal with more readily, if things were not so foggy. In fact, everything would have been more tolerable, had I been able to think clearly! Of course, one might be able to handle the affects of the near-electrocution better, if we didn't have to contend with other intrusions; those **"Added insults to injuries."** Yet, this is my life. My coping mechanisms are minimal, but I'm trying to find my way.

Some of life's little miseries were physical: As if I didn't have enough aggravation, I got my pants leg caught over a sprinkler head and fell; shattering my left shoulder and breaking the left elbow. My kids still say that I would not have fallen, if it were not for the delayed reflexes. I don't know; they could be right. Still, I think that spinning like a top, with arms out-stretched to regain my balance, was a perfect scenario for the dislocated (and shattered) shoulder and the fractured elbow. Sure, I've always been pretty active and agile, and I've taken spills before; but not like this. I think: *"First, lie still and assess the damage ."* You can pretty well guess things are not right, when you notice the elbow is bent in the wrong direction and your shoulder is sitting in front of you. Not a good sign! Lying there on my back, the pain was excruciating and I'm feeling faint and nauseous. (In the ER, we can usually tell if a child has truly broken a bone, before the X-ray results, if they are nauseous and faint. So, I'm a big kid. Everyone who has ever had a broken bone, says that the pain is unbelievable. Well, take it from me, you don't really know pain, until you experience a broken bone! Isn't childbirth worse? Right now, that's debatable!!)

Where is a neighbor when you need one?! Well, one is cutting the grass, another is edging his lawn, and the neighborhood basketball game is in progress out front. I could yell for help, against these odds or use my strength to shove the shoulder back in place; while rolling onto my stomach, with my right hand following the left arm down to the elbow and putting it back into the appropriate position, I rest. As painful as this was, the pain was a million times better, than before repositioning everything! Though you are weak and about to pass-out, you hope you have taken care of the compromised airway. (I had no choice but to take care of the situation, much as you would have to do, if this had happened on a hiking trail.) After about twenty minutes, I feel strong enough to get up. I splint my arm with a towel and drove myself to the ER. (WHY? It's that darn **20 Minute Delay** in assimilating information. I should have had a neighbor drive me to the ER, but they were all in the house having dinner, by now. So what? I should have had a neighbor drive me! I have great neighbors. Any one of them would have been glad to do so.) I was very thankful I had remembered to take the extra-strength analgesic before leaving home. X-rays completed, my elbow was immobilized with a half-open plaster arm splint and wrapped. The sling with an ice bag, relieved much of the pain; which is good, since I'm allergic to most pain medications. Acetaminophen is about the only thing I can use… even post-op.

Boy, was my husband surprised, when he got home from work. I sat in the recliner with my ice packs and the arm elevated on a couple of pillows. "Hi Honey, howww.." Yes, I know: "How was my day?" "A little more eventful than usual!" By the time I had finished at the ER, he had already left work. (If we had had cell phones, I could have cushioned the blow, somewhat.) Logic kicks in: What could he have done, seventy-five miles away? He would have just worried all the way home. He understands how I feel about *bugging people* needlessly. Just because I am miserable, is no reason to make others miserable. (That little tidbit, learned in childhood.) This would be a painful year of splinting, physical therapy, surgery, and more physical therapy. I should not lift anything over the head or sleep on the left side again. I will learn to work around that, though it will take ingenuity.

My younger brother, Carroll, would be relieved to know the Surgeon had not found a kneecap on my shoulder. As six and eight-year-olds, we practiced the instructions given us at school, for Fire Safety Week. I don't think they meant for us to practice an escape from a second story window that was twenty feet from the ground, but they hadn't made that clear. (These old farm houses were built on a three-foot berm, on top of a four-foot foundation, and the rooms had ten-foot ceilings.) However, practice we did. "Hang from the windowsill, push out with your feet (so you would clear the side of the house), and drop." My mother was busy fixing dinner and became curious when she noticed my brother and I were going up the stairs, but she hadn't seen us come down the stairs. Practice was over! (We never get to have any fun.) Someone had admonished us about how lucky we were that our kneecaps weren't sticking out of our shoulder blades. Sure, I had had the longer drop (counting the pad that the foundation was on), but my brothers room was over the concrete patio. That could smart! Amazing, isn't it? We were both past middle-age before we broke bones. It's a good thing. We would have missed out on all kinds of *FUN*, had we learned the pain of fun, while we were young.

Next, came the injury to the other shoulder. A very large patient flopped over on my hand while I was changing her bed. (Your reflex is to jerk your hand back; but, with three hundred pounds on your hand, it is not going anywhere.) Perhaps the delay in assimilation/reaction did play a part in this injury; not to mention the tennis elbows. This injury was to the right shoulder/neck/scapula/spine areas. Of course, I was cautioned to get help the next time. Sure! About 30 minutes is the limit I will let anyone lie in a wet bed. It is not as if you can leave the Cardiac Room and go on a hunting expedition. Either the help is there or it is not. I think, in the end, when all of the tests and bedrest was over, the final diagnosis was a stretched nerve (much like sciatica); with possible fraying of the superior rotator. (Give me a break! My *frayed nerves* are already *stretched to the limit*!) Whatever they called it, the spasms would leave you totally incapacitated; the pain was tremendous. Now, I have to *baby* this shoulder! I learned the hard way, I could not over-do work, using that arm. The spasms can cause a very painful distraction to your life, when they come along; much like sciatica of the neck, back, and shoulder. With my attention deficit, I really don't need any more distractions. So, now, both shoulders have the same lifting restrictions. I'll learn to work around it. Will someone be there to lift the IV bags for me? I doubt that. Who has time? I can use the step-stool. But, holding the cast-cutter at arms length, was impossible; even though, it only weighs eight pounds. That right arm is so weak and painful! No one really considers the affects of the injury on your work, much less anything else. (How about your swimming laps, carrying backpacks, mountain biking, scuba equipment, etc. Those little everyday pleasures, we take for granted. Even positioning for simple photography became a challenge. At my friends wedding reception, I looked like *The Hunchback of Notre Dame.*) Unless it happens to you, you can never understand. Why, we must lift our arms over our heads a million times a day! And though we are careful not to lift heavy objects at-arms-length, we lift smaller items all of the time. Even simple moves in dusting the furniture or washing a window, were too painful. These activities, all had to stop. Until I can regain some strength in that arm, everything is too heavy for me to carry and every job exerting pressure at-arms-length, is out of the question. It will get better, even if it never returns to normal.

When my husbands company "Locked-Out" the employees and he was suddenly out-of-work, we were pretty well tapped-out, financially. Three years before Eastern Airlines went under, we had invested in our retirement home. We put my retirement savings into a down-payment on the home we thought we would be spending the rest of our lives in. (This would make our house payments less, for our golden years.) It sure made sense, at the time. Are you listening to me? **Don't do that!** With my job, we could pay the bills for a while, but we would need both incomes eventually. With all of the resumes sent out, everyone interested in my husband, was in California. You might say, "The Handwriting Was On The Wall!" We were going to California!! He went to work for a large airline in San Francisco. We had enjoyed an A-1 Credit Rating our whole life. Even in our fifties, we would start-over! You say to yourself, that you are not the only people in the world, with these problems. We will do what we have to do. It's faith to reach out and Stubborn Determination to overcome the challenge! We can do this!

We were here less than six months, when my car hit a wheel in the middle of the expressway and was wiped out. (BUT, not me!) Even with our excellent credit rating, we could not afford new car payments, but could afford to lease a car. Lease payments are usually a hundred dollars a month less than new car payments; and often require no money down. We did the same thing with his gas-guzzling truck. (You will see the beauty in this indignity, later on.) As our automobiles would get close to the end of their lease, we still couldn't afford to buy-out the lease, so we would turn them in for a newer model. Everyone must have thought we were *in-the-money*; always driving new cars. They need not know why. If we could have afforded a ten year old model, that is what we would have been driving. It is only a mode of transportation, after all.

With that excellent credit rating and the equity in our retirement home, we were able to buy a house here. It would save some money in rent and we would not have to worry about finding another place, if the landlord wanted to sell. (They had been hinting that the family might like to move back into the rental house, to be closer to everything.) We bought a little house; all that we needed. Now, we could work on getting rid of our debts. After a while, we realized that the retirement home in Florida would have to go. We couldn't continue paying two mortgage payments, even with renters. We hated to do it. It was sort of like admitting defeat. (Or, was it facing the reality, that we had hung-on for too long?) We had pared-down so much already, we had hoped to keep our house.

My husband had sold his private plane, after loosing his job. He could always rent a plane. After we sold our retirement home, his father offered to help him get another little plane. My father-in-law felt that it was money his son would inherit one day anyway and he felt that he would like for us to enjoy it now. What a kind gesture! It sure lifted my husbands spirit! All work and no play … you know the rest. Of course, I could no longer concentrate on seven instruments at once, so I became a passenger instead of the Private Pilot I had been. Like I say, no one fully understands the changes that are brought about in a persons life, by a Company's carelessness and negligence. I still enjoy being up above it all; I just have to do it with another PIC. Most of the joy of flying came from the challenge of planning a trip and then setting it down on-the-numbers, right to the minute of the ETA. Now, that's an accomplishment! It does involve working out fourteen equations, before hand; but, it feels so good. (More of the little things we take for granted.) The Almond Blossoms are an awesome sight, come Spring. From the air, the whole valley is a mass of "pink snow." What a lovely world! Thanks to my husband, I can still enjoy this sight.

We were doing better, without the other house payment, so we were able to pay extra on our credit cards; we would have them paid-off in five years. (I know that may seem like a long time to some of you, but to us, it would be a dream come true.) Of course, *putting every extra cent into the credit cards* left us without savings for emergencies. **Don't do that, either!** Because, THEN, I lost my job. We had to consult a Bankruptcy Lawyer. They looked at our debt-load and said that the only thing they could suggest was Chapter 7 or a five percent pay-back on the dollar with a Chapter 11. Well, we were so indignant. We told the lawyer that we would just get a second mortgage on our home and pay off our bills. He was trying to tell us that our A-1 credit rating would no longer be viable, with our debt-load. We would find that out for ourselves. No mortgage company was interested in our A-1 rating with our debt-load and no equity in this new house. Reality Check! We no longer owned property in Florida… or much of anything, anywhere. We had to declare bankruptcy. What a disgrace! However, since we did not own the autos, they were not a part of the bankruptcy. (See? A blessing in disguise! We still had transportation; though, we still had those lease payments, also.) Good transportation is important in California. Everything is spread out. We spend hours on the roads. If we had spent more than fifteen minutes on the road, going to work in Florida, we would have been looking for another job. Boy, what happened to the leisure-time out here? Another rude awakening! Florida traffic is about as bad as California, now. Both, growing States.

You might have already guessed, my husband is the worlds very finest *Straight Man.* We have so much fun. Whatever would I do without my best friend? However, there is that ever present *Venus versus Mars.* I never really noticed how differently men and women perceive things. My husband and I know better than to try to explain how we are going to do something; we will come at a task from different directions, yet find the same successful conclusion. (I really hadn't given it much thought before.) You can pretty well bet that I am very glad to have my husbands help with any project I tackle now-a-days. And, I don't care what direction he is coming from. (You know, A.D.? **A**fter the **D**isability.) Of course, my brain still comes from the Venus angle. But, since my hands cannot accomplish the task anyway, my husband will help. We women know that *men don't know their own strength.* No matter what, don't ask him to help you put on your pantyhose. Your toes will be sticking out the end and it will take a very long skirt to cover the thumb holes in the legs. (I think, after I shattered my shoulder, I had determined that I would not be wearing pantyhose again. And everyone wonders why I wear jeans or skorts all of the time.) Let's face it, no matter how my husband attacks a task, it is going to be a better job than I could do, though I'm sure some of my projects are beneath him; you know, the macho man helping plant a flower bed. He always helps without complaints. Well, maybe some suggestions are a bit suspicious. "Do we really need a tree here? It will just be one more thing to edge around."

How can I go wrong spraying my ornamentals? Before he goes to work, he will double-check the amount of spray needed for the hose-end sprayer. I'll spray the plants this afternoon. We work together beautifully. I turned on the hose and opened the spray end. I (not the plants) was immediately saturated with fungicide. The hose had leaked around its metal fixture… not the washer. I jumped into the shower. Then, I called him at work to let him know what had happened. "Oh, yeah! I forgot to tell you the backyard hose needs new fittings." (Hey, we all make mistakes.) The next morning, I went to run an errand; the DMV was closed. I figured, as long as I was in the area, I could save my husband a trip to the hardware store. Let's see, he needed a couple of those florescent tubes for his shop light and a couple of hose fittings to repair the hose. I can guess the size of our hose, by looking at other hoses in the store. Proud that I had saved him a trip, I showed him my treasures. The light bulbs were fine; but, it seems, I bought the *wrong gender* hose fittings. Who would have guessed? Like buying a goldfish, how would you know? I had a doctors appointment that afternoon. I would exchange the *"females"* for *"males."* "Meanwhile, since you will have to cut the ends off anyway, why not do it now and I will take it with me for an example of the right gender and right od/id size?" He came into the house and handed me a piece of green hose-ending. I asked why he had cut off the green hose, when it was the gray one that leaked. "The green one doesn't leak?" he asked. "It does now." I replied. **Belly Laugh!** We will repair both hoses. (He thought I had said that the back yard hoses leaked… plural.) Maybe we should check our equipment each Spring, before using.

Our trees are getting big. It seems my husband thinks about selling the house when the trees get big enough for me to fall out of them…. I usually climb them and trim the branches myself. It's the Tomboy in me. He had witnessed one fall, of my sliding from branch to branch. "A lady your age should not be climbing trees." Doesn't he know: **Age, like IQ and MONEY are merely numbers; It's what you do with them, that counts.** One really has to figure in other factors, however. Perhaps I should stay out of trees, with my slowed reaction time.

* * * * * * *

Someone has to be a statistic. One in every seven women, over the age of thirty-five, will be diagnosed with Breast Cancer in their lifetime. I've always gotten the mammograms and GYN exams each year; and I do the SBEs every month, so the cancer was caught early. I remember awaking one morning, with a painful left breast. The important thing here is: this was something different; this was a change. It needed to be checked. Sure, I had found this little lump, on my monthly *self breast examination,* but it was hard to believe that something so small as half the size of a pea, could hurt so badly. I got right in to see my gynecologist. She couldn't find anything. I put her finger on the spot and was surprised she couldn't feel it between her finger and my chest wall. But then, it was very small, and **I** am feeling the pain of it being pushed against **my** chest wall. As she stated, "I don't really feel anything to be concerned with. You know," and I cut her off. I know the myth that cancer doesn't hurt, but I lost a friend to breast cancer thirty years ago, because her breasts were so painful. By the time she insisted that they remove them anyway, the cancer had spread everywhere. Still, the myths persist, to this day. **Let's get serious, here!** In Nursing School, I had a very wise instructor, who said, "In medicine, as in life, **THERE ARE NO EXCEPTIONS** TO THE RULES**, EXCEPT THE EXCEPTION** TO THE RULES**."** I was forced to insert this warning, when I heard a local TV doctor tell a call-in patient, "You shouldn't worry about it being breast cancer, if it is painful." I cannot allow this myth to be perpetrated on women. While cancer usually slips-up on us silently, there are always those exceptions. The presence of pain does not put you in-the-clear. (Mine hurt like a son-of-a-gun!) Nobody knows you, like you! If it is something different, check it out.

I was due my yearly mammogram the following month anyway, so she ordered it early. I dropped by the hospital and had the mammogram, then went shopping. When I returned home, there was a message from my doctor to "Call me right away." I called, and she said that I would have to arrange to have an open biopsy. There was something suspicious on my mammogram. I was given the doctors name and number to contact: "Classic Cancer!" Why did I cry? I had not felt that the gynecologist had taken me seriously. Often, doctors don't mean to be, but they are still condescending to women. Why not? Women are the worse offenders. i.e. I called the utility company to see if they had gotten my last check. "There are only two girls working in this office and one is out to lunch. You'll have to call back later!" Before I could ask her what the other girl was doing or how much later, she hung up. I hit re-dial and handed the phone to my husband. She was so sweet, the phone dripped of honey. She told him not to worry. The bookkeeper was on vacation and the postings were running late. She apologized for his inconvenience, and asked if there was anything else she could do for him. He thanked her for the information and handed the phone back to me. I thanked her for the information she had given my husband, but let her know that, "Until women start treating women equal, women will never be equal." (Please, women everywhere, feel free to quote me on that!) I think many of us have experienced similar situations. Let's not be a part of the problem. Be polite, but speak-up. And, let's check our own behavior.

I knew there was something wrong. (Woman's Intuition!) Confirmed by the mammogram. These are the same girls who do my mammograms every year. They had never brought me back for a second, (or a third) picture before. (Maybe, because I had been so adamant about finding something different, and "Intuition tells me, it is not the normal Cystic Breast Disease, 20 percent of we women feel, after bingeing on chocolate and other caffeine.") Like I say, someone has to be the statistic; but, let's get rid of the myths. We need not become victims.

It was a little discerning when they found something on the left lung. The **scar on the lung** could be a burn or from some undetected pneumonia. (Since infarcts are common in the soft tissues of organs, like lungs, kidneys, and liver, etc., I suspect the former.) I guess, I had just needed a good cry. It was scary, knowing that 27,000 more women died from lung cancer than died from breast cancer, in the year 2000. I had never smoked, but I do have an allergy to smoke; indicating that, perhaps, my lungs could have a problem from the second-hand smoke. 165,000 women a year, die from smoking-related disease. (Sure, "We've come a long way, babe!" But, who wants to die of lung cancer?) My nerves were shot, just waiting for the results of the current chest x-ray. However, upon closer examination of a previous chest x-ray, taken after the SHOCK, the shadow was there, AND it was determined, there had been no change.

I would have one surgery before Thanksgiving and another before Christmas. I had the open biopsy and lumpectomy, under local anesthesia. For a larger margin and removal of lymph nodes, I would go under general anesthesia. Everything went well and I had some pretty involved radiation therapy; after which, I was bothered with an encapsulated fluid build-up in the biopsy site (a seroma from the radiation-damaged tissue) This only happens in one out of every one-hundred. But, of course, I would be that one! It's the driving that is a bother; every week to ten days, I would go in to get it drained. I could hardly constrain the joy! (Oh, stop whining; they got rid of the cancer, didn't they?)

As a nurse, I am aware of the fact that the <u>number one killer of women</u> is still **Heart Disease.** 500,000 women will die each year, of this disease. (That is about twice as many as will die of all cancers combined.) We women have a tendency to take care of the rest of the family, and ignore our own care. It's time we start taking care of ourselves. Heart Disease is a real problem for women; because, we think it happens more to men and it's not a significant threat. What does that mean? More men? If 500,000 women die every year, something's wrong here. That is why the Surgeon General is suggesting that we watch our weight, eat a balanced diet, drink those eight glasses of water every day, exercise regularly, get plenty of sleep, stop smoking, and get regular check-ups and mammograms.

* * * * * * *

Before the cancer, we had decided to learn how to sail. My husband would learn the book work and I could learn from hands-on experience. I had taken the helm of a friends sailboat a couple of times and it felt just like flying *by-the-seat-of-your-pants.* The laws of physics never change: whether the airfoil is horizontal or perpendicular, fighting air currents above or water currents below, and watching wind direction to stay your course. So many of the same principles. We can do this! Along came cancer and we put it off for later. Later is now; the surgery is over. Now, let's talk about the angels among us. There was this little twenty-five foot sailboat for sale. A friend told us about it. (We didn't have "two nickels to rub together," but we felt we owed it to our friend to go look at the boat, anyway.) It was a great buy, but we didn't have the money. **A really great buy**, but we would have had to be late with the mortgage payment, to buy the boat. No way! There would be other boats.

A gentleman, with whom my husband worked, along with his wife (another nurse), wanted to give us the money for the boat; we could pay them back in a year or two, or whenever. When my husband told me about the offer, my first thought was not to accept. Then, the thought entered my mind that this was all too easy. Just maybe it was meant to be. You should always listen to that inner voice. My husband does deserve this exciting new hobby. It is something we plan on doing, someday.

I had been taught to always help others, while refusing help myself. We were taught self-sufficiency. i.e. I guess I must have been about five years old and my brother three. My mother was in the kitchen, fixing the biscuits for dinner. Some charitable organization brought a box of food to our door. When we said that our mother was busy, the man set the box in the middle of our living room, and was gone. My brother and I had never seen store-bought cookies, nuts, cereal, fruit and ham in a can, etc. We were into the candy and cookies, when our father arrived home from work. He made us put everything back and he took the basket back for *someone who really needed it*. Can someone be too proud?

He was right; we did have the usual chicken for Thanksgiving. My mother made great home-made egg-noodles and dumplings. There would be pickled peaches, in place of cranberry sauce. (We had canned several quarts). She would be making a fresh pumpkin pie and a raisin pie. Yes, it might not be the normal over-abundance of the typical Thanksgiving meals, but what I'd give for one of her meals today. We hadn't really needed the fancy store-bought vittles; we had plenty to eat. I realized later, that he did not want us to get used to something we could not afford. Once, when he was in the hospital a few days, he objected to we children staying with my city aunt; but, he had no choice.

While he was eating hospital food, we would be enjoying puffed wheat with canned milk. And we would get to help color margarine-in-a-bag, and enjoy other worldly things. To us, these were wonderful commodities. (Even "The Great Wall of China" can't keep out progress!) And to think, we had to endure fresh milk, churned butter, buttermilk, and cottage cheese instead of that canned milk. Hot oatmeal, cream of wheat, and cornmeal mush instead of the puffed wheat. My mothers biscuits, cornbread, and sweet rolls in place of store-bought bread. I can tell you, there was nothing better than my mothers sweet rolls with fresh-churned butter. The whole town could tell you that!

My father was an honorable and kind man, but was he really robbing people of the joy they could have received, from giving to others. Why had it taken me years to see that? I was just like my father. Guilty, as charged. You know what joy fills your heart, when you can help others. No one can explain that feel-good pleasure, but it's there. We never had money, but were taught that everyone has different talents. Use what you have: a smile and a kind word may be all that you have to give, but it will change some ones day; apples from your tree can make a nice pie for the neighbors; going to the store for that elderly gentleman; helping someone with their homework, will brighten their world and give self-esteem. So many things cost nothing, yet give joy and comfort. It always feels so good to help. Alright, we will accept the money for the boat. Just this once. We could not rob them of this joy. And, **they were so happy** to have helped. It looks like our "SOMEDAY" is today. We are beside ourselves, with joy!

The boat had belonged to a Minister. Parishioners had sewn curtains and covered the upholstery. (I keep telling everyone that this was a gift, straight from God; I can no longer make sense of sewing patterns or making pillow slips. The parishioners had already taken care of these things.) While it would take a lot of work before we sailed her, a lot of the work had already been done, or started. I just had to do cosmetic work (paint and clean), while my husband had to take care of the boat, motor, sails, lines, etc. We figured a good name for the boat would be The Bless-ed. It had received a lot of TLC from church people. It really was a blessing. (And, with such an honorable name, we could not resort to calling it other names, while working on it.) This boat was very effective in giving us something to think about; other than cancer and doctors appointments. It consumed our spare time. Though, I did have pretty good reflexes, when I christened the boat, it wasn't exactly *A Virgin using the bow.* More like, the bilge became my substitute bow. I was standing on the table painting the overhead, when I slipped and had a jarring-hard fall. Anyway, the boat was christened, without ill effects; good reflexes must be returning. I can find *positive* in anything! (Everything will be tested, in time. That good name we gave the boat came in handy. I never even thought a bad word.)

I can not thank the many compassionate people enough. Many have given us sailing hints. (We could not afford expensive sailing lessons.) We are learning to sail, but we learned a couple of important lessons for living, also. And yes, sailing really is like *flying by the seat of your pants.* We are having great fun. We really appreciate the help of the good people, who took us under their wings.

Thanks to all of our many friends. It sort of renews your faith in your fellow man. I am still receiving books as gifts, though I won't retain the information. I believe, many are getting the message; the books are usually short stories or short chapters, I can read for the pleasure of the day. I'm grateful to the gentleman who reminded me that I could have been like him: born without the ability to remember anything from one day to the next. (That will sure slap you out of any "Pity Party.") Thanks, I needed that! Many thanks to the complete strangers who put forth the effort to send me information, regarding the Electrical Current Burns. Since I cannot do research, these people would send me information, which was short and to the point, once they learned I was writing about the subject. I am grateful for each person who chose to make a difference. Most people are kind and good, loving and caring. I choose to see my world this way. How about you?

CHAPTER 15

I'VE COME A LONG WAY

I'VE COME A LONG WAY.

I've come a long way, in the past ten years. Do I know how incredibly lucky I am? You bet, I do! Six years after the Near-Electrocution, when the **FOG** lifted, I started taking back my control; or, as much control as one in this condition can exert. It's a slow process. With any success, comes a little more self-esteem. The "Can-Do-Girl" just has to find the things she can do!

Along with accepting my own disabilities and working with them, I've found new understanding in many other areas. The actions and reactions of those who do not understand and those who are trying hard to understand this challenge, are lessons unto themselves.

At first, I tried to conceal my condition; as if I could. I felt so damaged, so inadequate. With the slowed assimilation of material and slowed responses, I had lost that power to control my life. Whenever things were obviously in disarray, I would try to pull them together again; unwilling to accept the fact that I hadn't the power to do so. The frustration of responding slowly to a situation, finally prompted me to defend myself. I would have to admit that I had a problem; though, admitting to a **Shock**, may not be the way to go. Sometimes this was worse than the prejudged accusatory looks or words received, when I could not be my old self. I would say, "Oh, my words don't always come easily, since my **Electrical Shock**." It didn't matter that I used Electric<u>al</u> Shock. They would hear Electroshock Therapy. You could tell, people were automatically envisioning Frankenstein; wondering what I was doing out-of-the-hospital. I would hear such things as, "Bless your heart. We all have our problems, dear. As long as the shocks help, you'll do just fine." (I hope that wasn't a stab at encouragement!) Some, would just hurry away, faster than they had arrived; as if I had something contagious. What it all boils down to, there is a need to understand this condition. I would eventually add that I had received an Electrical Shock **from a faulty elevator.** One would hope that that would have been explanation enough. Think again! "Oh, My! Did that just happen? You should report it, before someone is seriously hurt." Then, they would go into great detail about everyone they knew, who had ever received a *buzz* from anything. You can see why I don't want to talk about it. I'm put-on-stage, to repeat the horror, over and over again. I'm trying to get-on-with my life. I needed a simple explanation, I could recite and brush aside. So everyone got the point, when I started calling it, like the doctors called it… a **Near-Electrocution**. No debate.

I've found that others will be willing to accept you, (in whatever condition), when you are willing to accept yourself. Though, admitting to a **Traumatic Brain Injury**, may not be exactly, the way to go, either. You may find a look of horror on their face, as they rush for the nearest exit. Like a broken bra strap, **we may be *defective,* but not dangerous!** While I get a 'kick' out of the funny episodes I've encountered from those who lack knowledge on the subject of brain injuries, it's time to educate. Once again, most of us fear things we do not understand. We can't run from our own ignorance. About half of America, isn't even familiar with the term "brain injury." How can this be, when we have 5.3 million Americans living with disabilities, which were the results of a brain injury? (50,000 die each year!) This means, that we must be mingling with them every day. They are nothing to fear!

While the results of a spinal cord injury may be easier to see, there are many, many more people with brain injuries. I'm sure you must recognize the fact that most of these injuries are caused by auto accidents, but there are many other causes, also: bikes, falls, strokes, near-drownings, drugs, lightening strikes, electricity, Sports related:(skiing a tree, falling from a horse, a bad football tackle, etc.), assaults, gunshot wounds, weakened or faulty construction and equipment; just to mention a few. Take caution! Don't ignore safety measures. Looking at these statistics, I no longer feel alone. I'm one of many. I can finally talk about my brain injury and the challenges I face; though, it is not my favorite pastime.

By Far, the greatest prevention of these types of brain injuries, is the use of seatbelts and bike helmets. Much as a pilot is responsible for the safety of his passengers, you, as the driver, are responsible for seeing that every occupant in your car is securely buckled into their seatbelt. Not only do these save lives, but they may prevent head injuries which lead to life-long disabilities. You need to set examples for your children.

There is nothing sadder than watching a family going for a bike ride; the children are wearing their helmets. We are pleased to see responsible parents, who are interested in preserving their children's lives. So, why is this a sad scene? Mom and Dad are not wearing helmets. (I'm here to tell you: a large head will split open, like a small head, when it impacts a curb.)

What happens, if Mom and Dad are no longer "there for them?" Shouldn't we be protecting the children's lifestyle, as well as their lives? Remember, **Children will be, what Children see.** I have this saying that may not be too popular, but it sure is real. "If you break a bone, we can usually fix it. If you break a head, _____?" The point is, generally, well taken. Forgive me, if I paused again, for another safety message; I am a Nurse!

So, we are living each day, among those who are physically or mentally challenged, due to a Traumatic Brain Injury. Some disabilities will be obvious, while others may go undetected. Some of these injuries will be the result of contact with electricity. Be patient and be compassionate. There, but for the Grace of God…

While brain injuries differ, some methods of assistance remain the same. Some family members are embarrassed or ashamed, when they should know that there is no reason to be. (Would you believe, many victims of brain injuries, feel the same way? We are often embarrassed or ashamed of things we cannot control. We feel like, if we just try a little harder, the wrong words wouldn't come out; or perhaps, we should be able to express ourselves better. After all, it's been ages, since the accident! BIG TIME DENIAL! We do not always control these things. Sometimes, they choose to control us. It is better, if everyone accepts the truth, looking to an improved future; no matter how long it may take. For some of us, improvement comes from learning to work-with what we have.) No one is prepared for an accident. It happens to someone else. When it happens to you, or someone close to you, you're in denial. It takes a while to grasp the reality, and turn the anger and frustration into concern and compassion:

You might hear some parents talk about the young man, who has had a brain injury; and is now screaming, hitting, kicking, and using four-lettered words they don't even recognize. The parents are apologizing to the staff. "Our son was never raised that way. I don't know what has gotten into him! He's never acted like this!" Of course, he's not himself. He's had a brain injury! Believe me when I say, the staff is used to brain injuries and their reactions. No apology needed. Still, by letting us know that this behavior is something highly unusual, may help us prioritize procedures, in order to speed his diagnosis and care.

When Mama has a stroke and her gibberish doesn't make sense, you may be tempted to say, "Oh, she's talking crazy. Don't pay any attention to her. She doesn't know what she's saying." Would it help, if I told you Mama probably understands everything that is being said? Can you even begin to imagine how frustrating it would be, not being able to express yourself?

How about, "Dad is just getting old. He has trouble remembering anything, since his by-pass surgery." There may have been a lack of oxygen, during his surgery. Don't dishonor him. Help him regain his dignity. He is probably aware of everything that is going on.

Just maybe, inside these heads are the same people as before, who are merely unable to express themselves appropriately. Just because they cannot express themselves, doesn't mean they are vegetative. Talk to them, in a normal tone. Unless they are hard of hearing, don't raise your voice. A normal conversation, spoken distinctly, will be appreciated. PLEASE, skip the *Baby Talk,* also. Speak to them, age appropriately. Many possess the same IQ as before the accident, and will be using that IQ to train other parts of their brain, to do the tasks the opposite side has forgotten. Be patient, when they try to speak; let them know that you appreciate their effort. And, encourage them **to keep on, keeping on.** This attitude tells them a lot. It gives them hope and it tells them that you care. Both, vital for any recovery.

Many are out there with permanent brain damage, which is only a challenge; not the end of their life. I guess you may have wondered why Mama was so cool to you, once she learned to talk again; and Dad is re-writing his will, after recovering from the surgery. (They probably remember your planning their funeral or fighting over the inheritance, while at their bedside.) While some may not have a recovery, how would you know who will or how many will not? Let's use The Golden Rule. I wouldn't plan the funeral or discuss who gets what possessions, in front of *the brain injury patient*. They just might rise to meet the challenge! (I can think of nothing that would make me more determined to recover, than a family fighting over my will. Unless, of course, I had a family genuinely praying for my recovery!)

People want to know,
WHERE AM I , NOW?

If someone is attempting to *get-on-with-their-life*, they must accept reality. We learn to work-with the "Whole," and adjust to the holes. (That would be the holes in our abilities.) It took ten years for me to stop playing games and admit to my brain injury. It's a sign of growth, when one can overcome the false pride of embarrassment, as you say or do something *off-the-wall*. Do you know what? I've learned to roll-with-the-punch, as they say. I can admit to anyone, I have an occasional problem with my speech; so, when I have problems finding the words, it is just a dropped chip in the old computer, from my Near-Electrocution. (Otherwise, how could you explain a woman being at a loss for words?) Believe it or not, people are always kinder, when you are willing to level with them. I've had perfect strangers playing "Twenty Questions" with me. It's a hoot! We laugh about it, but at the same time, I'm being successful in letting people know about Electrical Burns.

Most people I've met, have accepted me for who I am. I would wish the same for others, suffering from brain injuries. (Though, I must admit, I am still a bit perturbed by my loss-of-words or not being able to explain something I know perfectly well. I'm sure, there are many who share my problem. I know I can't help myself, but that *perfectionist* in me, doesn't like it.) Most days, my conversation is fluid. When it goes haywire, I'm frustrated; but I feel compelled to just make-light-of-it. You may as well laugh; it has become a-way-of-life. It's a way of coping. With humor, nothing is quite as bad as it was perceived. The same holds true for my typing. Occasional misspelled words, don't bother me. It is when all of the letters become juxtaposed, that I know it is time to *call-it-a-day.* Yes, I've learned to laugh about it. Besides, juxtaposed letters look funny; like a foreign language, or some secret code. Just try to keep a straight face! The Grin*ch* is in. Choose one!

I'm luckier than a lot of brain injury patients. My deficits are, for the most part, things you can learn to cope with. Your best tool in coping, will be accepting reality. You really must learn to laugh at yourself, because that *Sophisticated Lady* is going to say and do some pretty silly things. A shoulder shrug is always a good explanation. Then, look sheepish. (People will expect, and accept, anything from a blonde.) The *Lady* may not wish to go into details, while at a party.

They say that, if you're married long enough, you'll finish each others sentence. That may be true. I've seen it often enough. Well, my husband is a genius; he knows what I mean, before I spit-out the words. Fortunate? Of course, but **he** just **knows me!** (Too bad he can't finish my thoughts.) On the days, when every sentence starts with *lost words* or *lost thoughts,* he will start a subject of his own; then, I can join in. What a gentleman! He does protect my dignity.

The **20-Minute Delay** (or whatever we are calling it this week,) is a real nuisance! A reliable answer to any involved question, can take twenty minutes, in the least; sometimes months. Simple "Yes" or "No" questions, much sooner; maybe, five to ten minutes! You should never expect accurate answers, until the slowed processes are given the time to consider all aspects. **On a good day**, you might get a quicker answer; though, it may not be the one I would give, 4 months from now. And, on the really good days, none are the wiser. **On a bad day**, I wouldn't rely on any answer. Fortunately, **BAD DAYS ARE FEW!** Hints are often helpful; Suggestions are expected and accepted. Thanks!

Just **coping, with the coping** of a brain-injured person, can be challenging:

Say, you and your husband are busy cleaning the garage, when you realize it is 2:00 and you haven't had lunch. He offers to go through the drive-in of the local burger joint and get us some take-out. "What do you want?" "Oh, I don't care; anything will do. Just get me a grease-burger." As soon as he drove out of the driveway, I'm wanting to change my order. I never eat grease-burgers! I guess I will today. You really need to help me here. Offer suggestions. Would I like a grease-burger, a half-dozen chicken nuggets (at 80 calories each), or a grilled chicken sandwich? That would be a quick and easy choice.

Like I say, on my more fluid days, no one is the wiser. I seem perfectly normal. Most days are like that. I LOVE FLUID DAYS! On those rare days, when nothing is working right (so it seems to me), one would be tempted to stay home. **You can't win a battle, if you are not willing to enter the fight.** Sometimes, it will be a very tough fight, but the victory is so sweet. Defensive Practice, gives one added confidence. Like I say, most days are "*Normal*," some are "*Challenging*," and some, are "*the Devil on your back*!"

I have a haircutting appointment this afternoon. I will pick up the dog's Heart Worm Prevention medication at the Vet's; it's on the way. I write myself a note and put it on the stirring wheel, so I won't forget. I'm not that sharp, today! (We must have low barometric pressure.) Well, that only took a moment. I grabbed the pills and my receipt and.... and run for my car. I know I parked close. Where is that car? I'm walking up and down the lane of cars, when I realize I had been looking for a white car. I've had the new car for three months, now. I still don't see that dark-green car anywhere. Did someone steal it that fast?! I can always walk the two blocks to the hairdresser's, but I will have to report my stolen car first! In total frustration, I take off my sunglasses, leaning against this car, parked in my space! Oh, no! I am standing right next to a dark-green car, which had appeared black, with my sunglasses on. Reality catches up with me and I wonder: How could anyone steal that car? It is like Ft. Knox! (All of those new futuristic Keys with a Chip, ***GPS equipment,** state-of-the-art Alarms, etc.; you name it, these new cars have it all.) This *Detective* is very relieved! It would have been so embarrassing to report a car missing, while I'm standing right next to it! I opened the door and tossed the dog pills and my receipt onto the passenger seat. If I hurry, I will be on time for my salon appointment. Arriving on time, I went in and had my haircut. I'm relaxed now! Nothing like a shampoo and cut to relax a harried soul.

How fortunate I am, to have this ***little green car that looks black***. I can not say enough about **The Lady in the Box.** Lexus, and Camry came out with this particular type of miracle... my simple GPS System that can take you to any address; no guessing. I just put in the address and "The Lady in the Box" takes me there. She will tell you how far it is, how many miles you have before making a right (or left) turn, how long it will take to arrive, etc. I mean, how simple can that get?! We drove four thousand miles cross-country without looking at one map. She took us from our doorstep to their doorstep in record time. But, just like instrument flying, you have to learn to trust the Lady. She may use some back roads; a short run North, even though you are heading East; skirt busy expressways; or take several shortcuts through back streets and residential areas to avoid stop-and-go traffic. However, "The Lady" has never been wrong. I cannot tell you how much time and anxiety that can save someone with Attention Deficit and Short-Term Memory. This came in real handy, when we moved to another town.

Well, no looking for the car this time; it is right out front. I opened the door and got in; BUT wait, what happened to the dog pills with the receipt I had left on the passenger seat?! Oh, no! In my hurry, I must not have locked my car. Now, someone has my credit card number. I will need to notify the bank; but, what about identity theft? **What a day this has been!!** It all has to do with **That 20-Minute Delay!** (Actually, some days are worse than others. When I say I am not so sharp, that means that my delays in assimilation are extended, to one degree or another.) No need to fret about it. I can't do anything until I get home anyway. Before I call the bank about canceling my credit card, I'll check with the Vet's office. (With my Short-Term Memory; maybe I hadn't brought the stuff to the car, in the first place.) Let's make sure I hadn't left them on the counter, at the Vet's. "No, I hadn't left them there. She thought she saw me put them in my bag." Alright, so I did take them with me. I'll check the car once more; maybe I put them under the seat, before I went into the salon. Well, they are not under the seat and they are too big to fit into the console or glove box... (I haven't changed modes yet; my brain is still putting out information on my former car). Ah, I do like this new car. It has two consoles; a nice flat one over a deeper one. This is so great! You can keep the boat key and gate card in the shallow console and put bigger stuff in this nice deep console... like these dog pills and the receipt!!! God knows! Sometimes I *overwork* this investigative job! Maybe, I just needed a little stimulation. Right now, I need a little mental rest; put on the music, call a friend and laugh about it all. Let's remember to Thank God for the abilities we do possess. Yes, I'm glad I can still *put-the- pieces-together*, no matter how long it takes. I'm much better at accepting, that this is just a part of me; I'm hoping others understand. This *detective work* is on-going. This had just been one of those Super Frustrating Days, when **nothing seemed to be working right!** In a short time, I will be looking for that little green car every time, instead of the white car. Like the Large Letter Edition books, I will enjoy the assets that come my way.

In this condition, I am constantly scanning my resources, looking for coping mechanisms that might work. You never know when you might stumble onto a new solution. The Large Letter Edition magazines helped with my reading enjoyment, but that only solved one aspect of the problem. I must rely on others to come up with some solutions. When I think someone else might have a solution, I'm not too proud to beg.

In my teens, we would visit the "Old Folks Home" and help the elderly to church services. **They would put-you-to-shame!** I don't care how senile or infirm they were, they always sang their hymns with gusto. Experiencing the Love these elderly showed, while worshipping their God, was inspiring. We teens were reminded again that our songs of praise were not for the congregation, but for the Lord. None of us would ever hold-back again. As the years rolled by and we moved from one town to the next, I didn't quite feel I was participating in worship, as fully as before. Many churches had gone to an over-head projector, to supply words to "Row Songs" for the people to join in. How does one sing without the notes? I longed for the good old days; and, I'm not even that old. I had so much difficulty with the *row songs*, and couldn't understand why. On special Holy Days, I had renewed joy in my heart. I felt that my worship was complete. There were the traditional songs of the Season, that's why. How could I expect to remember something flashed before my eyes? With my Hand/Eye Coordination messed-up, I could not follow words on an over-head screen. With the Short-Term Memory, I'm certainly not going to remember words to "Row Songs" from one week to the next. Since there are so many people with Brain Injuries, how about throwing in a *Golden Oldie* each week? Perhaps some up-lifting song of our Religion's Faith, Hope, Love, and that Joy of inner Peace that surpasses understanding. We "*Have Faith in God"* because "*God Will Take Care of You*," so "*Revive Us Again." "Pass It On,"* and *"Let there Be Peace On Earth."*

Some instances leave you with a whole array of your disabilities exposed. You will be facing those more complex delays, on occasion: The Doctor explains what tests he will need, but his secretary will arrange the appointment. So, she forgot. I put the date on my calendar; the lab can always call the doctors office and find out what tests he needs. I know he always requires a fifteen-hour fasting, also. At my next doctors appointment, the Doctor will go into minute details about the tests and the results. Will I remember? No. (I'm still the one with Short-Term Memory.) **Write it down, please!** Better yet, send home a copy of the laboratory results. I can then study them at my leisure; and refer back, when needed. Most doctors have learned, but they have so many patients, I may have to remind them, on occasion; and, they don't mind. In fact, may appreciate it. Get ready! The embarrassment never stops, unless you refuse to let it *get to you*. In my files, I can see reports of Lab Work, MRI's, Stress Tests, Cardiac Caths., Surgeries for one thing or another, etc., BUT, I don't remember them! (I guess there is something to be said about Short-Term Memory! … Unless your doctor asks when you had your last EKG, and you advise him to "Check my file.") In these ten years I've spent teaching my Doctors to be my advocate, my life has become so much easier. Finally, anything seems possible; *THEN*, we moved far away! (I must now, start all over again!)

Maybe I've become too complacent with my doctors. Even if I had to remind them occasionally, they worked with my Short-Term Memory. It is not easy for anyone to find new doctors in another town, but with my many problems, it was twice as difficult. I know, you are thinking that you will wait until you're moved-in and settled before you start your search. Nah, it doesn't work that way. I can almost guarantee, someone will have an earache, toothache, broken finger, turned ankle, irregular pulse, bronchitis, a strange new mole, a breast lump, a head bump, up-set stomach, or just be up-set. Let's see, did that cover all specialties? So you find yourself checking out strangers smiles and asking about their dentist; checking haircuts, and asking "Who does your hair?" While in the ER with your kid and the broken finger, ask about a good dermatologist, cardiologist, gynecologist, etc., (and you could probably use a good psychologist, by now.) It's rough fending for yourself in this **Big Strange New Location.** Like I've said, I'm not too proud to ask for help. With my hand full of new doctors and their addresses, I can just leave the task of finding them to my *Lady in the Box*. Still, other obstacles await!

O.K., now that you have found your batch of doctors, make copies of your families' vaccination sheets, list of allergies, medications taken, surgical procedures and latest lab reports, etc. This way, you can just pass them from one office to the other. Just write "See Attached" on those office forms everyone has to fill out. This is especially helpful for those of us with Carpal Tunnel Syndrome; and, your hands will *quietly* thank you! (Who knows, you may get home in time to go through a few of those boxes you still have to unpack!) With my Hand/Eye Coordination messed-up, it takes me forever to read and separate the tiny lines of faded print, on **the usual office forms**. A recent batch I was handed, even had one printed cater-cornered. That did it! PLEASE! I have enough obstacles to overcome. I took it up to the receptionist and told her I couldn't read it; it's too difficult for my *Hand/Eye Coordination.* (That went over her head!) She looked at me as if she understood I was illiterate and compassionately explained what the form said; then asked me to sign it. *Changing Modes* from subject to subject can be very tiring, also. It's a long frustrating process for me: I arrive before the appointed time, and am still filling out forms when the doctor is ready to see me... then, they are waiting for me to finish. Meanwhile, all of the later appointments have gone ahead of me. I think we all need a lunch break! At any rate, by the time I actually see the doctor, I'm *used-up*; my brain needs a rest. All of the problems and questions I had been prepared to ask, were now forgotten and my appointment had been just a huge monumental waste of time. By now, I am like a brainless robot; the Doctor asks the questions and I answer the questions, *to the best of my ability.* (And the notes of questions and problems I had brought with me, are still in my pocket. I forgot to take them out.)

(So, even confessing my problems in advance, did little good. I was told, "That's alright, we will be glad to help you." Silly me! I actually believed that! How did she help? She gave me a clipboard with six forms to fill out, and a pen to write with. **Confessions help little, without <u>their</u> full comprehension.** "Why hadn't I reminded her, I'd need help?" Perhaps, because of the Attention Deficit or Short-Term Memory. I will remember that little fact, while I am driving home.)

The new doctors will ask you about any surgeries you may have had in the past ten years or any health problems they need to know about. My stock answer is always, "No. I'm healthy as a horse." (As I change modes…) "Well, I did have a cholecystectomy. I think that might have been in the past ten years; but then, **<u>You have a list of everything</u>.**" The new Doc sees that I have a problem; which means, HE HAS NOW, inherited that problem. Then, he looks at my Medical Records with the various operations, tests, and allergies. He realizes he has just received a Very Big Problem! (Most doctors are too busy to even phantom spending all of that time on one patient. Hey, but that is why they have assistants; to assist.) So, we start all over again, and I tell him about the Near-Electrocution <u>first</u>. Why can't I just walk in and say that *I am challenged*, right up front? Because my manners tell me that we should get the introductions and pleasantries out of the way first; then Attention Deficit kicks in, and I forget. (Especially, if he is busy asking me about what medications I'm currently taking; I'm on a mode change.) Sorry!

So now, I admit to my challenge up-front. You would think that would help. It doesn't. It goes right over their heads. I tell you, **I look too *normal* and sound too *normal*** (most of the time); until we get into particulars. Now, I realize that this is just another problem I'll have the rest of my life. Learn to accept and live with it. Perhaps **I should print up cards** explaining the extent of my Slowed Assimilation to Stimuli, the on-going Attention Deficit and my Short-Term Memory (which is usually, lost over-night). We do the best we can to cope with our challenges, in order to preserve our dignity and to live a better quality of life.

Printed Info Cards might help!

(Then again, maybe not.)

While you have seen examples of my symptoms throughout this book, I wonder how you would cope with a few of these problems. Simple everyday things we take for granted, become our greatest challenge. You may spend the rest of your life looking for solutions that don't exist. That doesn't mean you stop looking. Futile, with Short-Term Memory? Perhaps, but I keep trying. What chance do you have of developing new friendships? I'm a friendly sort of soul, up-beat and happy. I have a lot of fun. Meeting others has always come easily, for me. Maybe, because I love people, and find every one interesting. They all have fascinating stories to tell. I've met great people, from all walks of life. Many with whom, I feel I could become close friends; however, those fabulous interactions of today, are gone in the night. With Short-Term Memory, I go to sleep and yesterday is forgotten. (I wonder what my History Teacher would say about that! Probably, "You have brain damage! Too bad you couldn't have used that excuse before.")

Alright, so I was still embarrassed by some happenings: People smile and speak to me on the street, like some long-lost friend, "Hi! How are you?" "I'm doing great. How are you?" (When I really want to say, "Who are you?") I can always chat about the traffic, weather, clothes, etc., while waiting for a hint. *She is so nice, but who is this person?* With the Short Term Memory, our lovely two-hour conversation (about tropical plants, extended families, upcoming concerts, robotic flies, or whatever), in the doctor's waiting room, had been forgotten long ago. Would you say, "Give me a hint. Where have we met? Tell me again, what we were talking about, 'cause I forgot." **That should win friends and influence people!** Presenting your name, where we met, and the subject of our conversation may jar some memories. If not, let's try again. I may not have total recall, so I'll depend on your cognition. Fortunately, repetition does help my recall. Shouldn't everyone be required to wear compulsory name tags at all public meetings? (I could only hope, but it might be a bit Orwellian, to expect that.) I do appreciate the ones who wear name tags, at church.

If you pass me on the street and I act like I don't know you, I'm not being rude. I probably don't know you, if I haven't seen you for a while. Don't feel dejected. Know that the same holds true for some renowned Surgeon, who has just done wonders for my health; I only saw him for consultation, pre-op, post-op and follow-up. Though he did great work and had terrific bedside manners, I wouldn't recognize him, if I passed him in the hall. He is probably thinking that I am some ungrateful snob. (When you think of it, a woman seldom talks to a *Strange* Man.)

I do remember most of my neighbors, whom I see frequently. That is a blessing! (However, if they are away on extended vacation, I may not recognize them, when they return. Once again, repetition will help.) I would love knowing some of the other people I've met. So, go ahead, give me a hint. I really wouldn't be embarrassed, if you reminded me of your name and where we met; maybe, we'll be able to continue the conversation, we were having then.

Most don't even know that I have this problem. **I guess you will understand, if you are reading this book.** *You encourage us, to keep trying.*

I'm here to say that there are fabulous people all around us. We need to take the time to listen to them. I may not become a lasting friend, but I enjoyed your up-lifting conversation. Did you spark a delightful memory of my childhood? Sure, I can remember when my babies or children did the same thing, yours are doing now; and, it brings laughter and wonderment of the fact that kids remain the same. They still try the same old tricks my kids pulled, and their parents pulled before them. **I WANT TO THANK YOU! (You see,** without ever knowing it, **you have helped someone through another day.** Your generous input to a casual "Good Morning," has given us the gift of socializing. A simple smile tells us we are a part of the whole; this whole world community. Strangers laughing together over silly observations, is so special. Keep it coming!) Thank you!

* * * * * * *

Just For-The-Day

Though my fun is just-for-the-day,
I will not give that fun away.

Thankful for the journey, I'm given.
Learning to live with the one, I'm skin in.

Looking for the joys, big and small,
Makes life more precious, to one and all.

What would I wish for everyone?
Peace, Happiness, and a Heart-Full of Song.

* * * * * * *

No one loves little children, more than I. My *Attention Deficit* caused another problem, I had not anticipated: I could not tolerate the presence of a lot of excited children, all trying to talk to me at once. (Back to that part about **changing modes**, to set your watch. With the slowed assimilation of the material being received, I am left behind; "O*ut of the Circle*." Though, it is really just nano-seconds, so most people would not detect the problem, I have to adjust to any new situation. It is still a matter of moving my thoughts and responses along; something that comes naturally, to the normal person. **While some people have mood changes, I have "mode changes."** I have to change modes, in order to go into a new subject of conversation.)

A bunch of children, talking all at once about separate subjects, was overwhelming, to me. I'd come home from the party, in a daze. Finally, my husband says, "I don't know why you put yourself in these situations. Don't attend parties with a lot of loud, interrupting children." But, I love children! And, I love being around them! "Well, maybe this is one of the things you will have to sacrifice; at least, the length of time you spend with them. (Or, wait until they are older and calmer.)" He grins! He's right, of course. I have no trouble talking with them, one-on-one. For every problem, there is a solution; but first, you have to acknowledge you have the problem.

These things I used to do, and can no longer participate in, are (once again) frustrating. I needed to Chill-Out! It is not the end of the world! The kids were running the show. Now, that's funny! I can't believe I bought-into their Attention Deficits! If I were not so slow *on the up-take*, I could have simply said, "One-at-a-time, Please. We cannot hear anyone, if everyone talks at once." Yes, I miss not being as quick and sharp, as before.

After all these years, I'm still grappling to ***find-my-way, day-to-day.*** I do try to read the morning paper; something that would normally take 20-30 minutes, now takes 2-3 hours. The lines of print are indistinct, small, and they run-together. (Even with my Apraxia of Hand to Eye Coordination, I still feel a need to accomplish this *little fete*!) Futile? Perhaps, but it's my way of **keeping on, keeping on!** When the papers start stacking-up, I have to go ahead and toss them anyway. For one who was used to reading three newspapers a day, I found this *compulsion* so incredibly strong. Again, thinking if I just try a little harder, I'll get better. Perhaps it's time for me to admit **this is <u>never</u> going to happen!** (Like my Neurologist used to say, "This was not a simple brain injury; there had been brain damage.") Through the years, I'm still finding areas of DENIAL, <u>needing my acceptance</u>. Sometimes, others will accept my disabilities, better than I.

There will always be situations that throw-me, when least expected. The difficult part, is recognizing the situation, as a "Situation." Perhaps, learning to accept and working with the Slowed Mode should be a goal?! Can that work? Maybe… if I didn't go to sleep. Like I've said, "Tomorrow is a brand new day." I will be seeking solutions again, in that *Brand New Day.* Sometimes, my husband will remind me of a better method of doing something, which he had observed before. This helps. (Remember the food chopper?) Still, there is Venus and Mars!! I'm doing better, in that respect (I tell myself); but it is just deductions and conclusions: Good Detective Work. I wanted to surprise my husband with a cake (we seldom have rich desserts), but there was one draw-back; we don't have an electric mixer and stirring by hand 200 strokes, will be too painful for my Tennis Elbows. Deductions: What have I ever made that might have required the use of an electric mixer? Let's think. Waffles! Conclusion: Yes, I must have a mixer, someplace. I start looking and find the mixer. I suppose you can say, I'm more independent now. That feels good. I think, "Promising."

(So, why am I still looking for the silverware, every morning?)

How many times would you find the word "Love" in the Bible? Now, how many times will you find the word "Frustration," when we describe our disabilities? Both words, countless. We don't like to talk about our frustration, but it's there. (Trying to read that morning paper was a real study in frustration! It had always been a relaxing routine; eat your breakfast and read the morning papers. When this "Can-Do-Girl" can't do it fast enough or good enough, why did I keep trying? Old habits are hard to break? I don't know. Maybe because I found it so relaxing, ***when I stopped!*** Accepting my problem as permanent, could relieve the stress of constantly striving for the impossible. So, I have learned to limit that *compulsion* to 20 or 30 minutes, a few times a week; if I miss something important, "Oh, well." I have better things to do. (Reality Check: I plan to sleep nights, so I won't remember what I've read that day, anyway; that's why I keep a folder of clippings. Still, some things are retained; and are *spit-out* when least expected.)

It can't be easy for the caregiver, either. Both need friends and relatives to lovingly prod us about these feelings, so we can talk about them. Caregivers have frustration over watching our failures, then listening to our frustrations, while encouraging us to keep trying. It is never healthful for either, to keep anything pent-up. (Let us know that you understand what we are going through, and that you are there to help, in any way that you can. We will appreciate that.) So, I've learned: It really isn't the End of the World, you know!

Love can overcome frustration. Remember, we are not that unusual, after all. There are those other 5.3 million Americans, living with the disabilities attributed to Traumatic Brain Injuries! We are just one, of millions. If they can do it, so can we.

Though I hadn't planned on it, this ***detective work*** has become a big part of my life. It certainly keeps one busy! This probably stimulates my brain better than sitting around doing nothing. (I even enjoy watching mysteries; challenging myself to solve the cases.) Whatever it takes to make the most of my abilities, I'm going to try. I may not find faster assimilation of material, but ***my life is more interesting***, simply ***fighting to live it.*** So, go on; live each day to the fullest, <u>that you</u> possibly can.

Suddenly, I awakened and there was bright sunlight, beating in through my window. Oh no! I had had an early doctor's appointment and would have to drive in the rush-hour traffic. I had set my alarm, but it must not have gone off. I will have to call the doctors office, apologize, and set-up another appointment. As I throw back the covers, I notice that I am fully dressed. I glance at the clock and it reads 3:00. I must have already gone to the doctors. Naturally, I would be dead-tired and in need of a catnap. I looked in my purse and saw a new prescription, so there is no problem, (except my *Short Term Memory*!) I guess I had needed more than just a little catnap. I had gone into a sound sleep, so I hadn't remembered my day's activities. Just as well; rush-hour traffic is wild. This is one of those little things that would have been embarrassing, had it happened elsewhere. It doesn't bother me any more. I can usually deduct what is happening, eventually. The detective work keeps me on-my-toes. I have to use my brain more thoroughly, and be more intent. Those *Rogue Roads,* with the ruts of scarred pathways, are becoming well traveled; perhaps, straightening some of the curves, thrown my way.

I understand my challenges, and have learned to live with most of them. Every chance I get, though, I step-up and take back my power. I had needed a good nap, after the daunting drive today, (not to mention the **Stress Echocardiogram**, I see scrawled across my wall calendar). As I retraced my activities of the day, I understand why I am so tired. With the facts before me, I can take charge of my destiny right now; by going back to bed!

"WE MAY BE DEFECTIVE, BUT NOT DANGEROUS!"

CHAPTER 16

MY RE-EVALUATION.

MY RE-EVALUATION.

As you read the pieces of my life BC, did you wonder why I included these memories of the past? We could say that this is all I have, but really, my cup runneth over. I have enough wonderful memories to last a lifetime and a half. I am so grateful for this wonderful life. The memories I have are precious. I rely on my family and friends to remind me of the present. (They have some pretty great memories, also.)

I have my childhood: My little brother and I eating the green grapes. (one of those interesting things we learned while staying with the city aunt, when Daddy was in the hospital.) I mean we saw people eating green grapes in the grocery store; our concords were usually purple. So they are smaller and green; they must be ready to eat. I wonder if those people in the store know that they will have to take a lot of castor oil for their tummy aches. Should I even mention jumping off of the henhouse with towels tied around our necks. How does Superman do that? We even tried jumping from the hayloft. That pile of soft mud below, broke our fall. Well, maybe it wasn't really mud; they had just shoveled out the stalls. Now that I have children of my own, I understand that look of "disbelief" my Mother often wore. The memories of my childhood, are of a Mother with "eyes wide open" in wonder. As we grew older, it would always be a smiling Mother, with pure "sweet serenity."

Visiting our Grandmothers house every summer, was the greatest thing that could happen to my cousin and me. Even if we had to spend a lot of time in the corner, while we were there; it was worth every moment. She would pick us up in her Rumble-seat car, and, we would become glamorous Hollywood Stars in our chauffeur-driven convertible, with wind blowing through our long hair. When we hit the old rutted country roads and lanes, our jungle entourage was obviously being carried by our guides, or we were riding on top of elephants. This was a great way to start our Summer! On the farm, there was so much space. We needed a lot of wide-open spaces, after being cooped-up in school for nine months. We found this one, especially beautiful, field to explore. It was big enough to build separate playhouses. We just stomped down the grass to make the walls of our house. When we finished stomping down the walls and dividing the rooms, we needed furniture. We remembered the big rocks along the fence line. We rolled them into place and started playing house. Here comes Grandma, with a switch. We didn't do anything. We're not hurting anything. She made us roll all of the rocks back to where we had found them. It was time for a long stay in the corner. So, what had we done so wrong, this time? It seems we had picked the alfalfa field. See, Crop Circles have never been a mystery to us!

(We did get a better education in those two weeks at Grandmas, than the nine months we spent in school. In Grandmas corners, we were captive audiences. Our Grandmother was a Women's Libber. Need we say more?)

Then, there were the swimming holes we played in, on those hot summer days, while riding our bikes. I never said we knew how to swim, only that we played in the swimming holes. One we especially liked, was a waterfall over a smooth rock. It was so much fun! (Like a slippery-slide ride.) Of course, it was very deep right under the fall, but we figured we could always hold our breath long enough to walk to shallower water. We had the same confidence, playing in the boys dammed-creek swimming hole. We were careful, though. Only one of us jumped in at a time. The other stood by with a long stick for the *swimmer* to grab, just in case. Our theory was the same for diving into the public swimming pool. We couldn't swim, but we figured we could hold our breath long enough to walk to the side of the pool and hang onto the side, walking hand over hand, until we reached shallow water. Life Guards, are you paying attention? We learned to dive beautifully, before ever learning to swim. We had great "form" and practiced "cutting the water" just right. Why, we were regular Esther Williamses.

I absolutely idolized my big brother, much to his disdain. I followed him everywhere. I was so sure he wouldn't mind, my taking his car for a spin on Highway 66, **when I was twelve**. (Well, I wasn't so sure that I would ask him first.) Besides, my cousin said we would just take it around the block; we could bring it right back and park it in the same place. No one would even miss us. Sounded good to me. *Around the block* included a steep hill. Going down the hill was no problem; I could see fine, even if the brakes were a little hard for me to hold down. Going up the hill was a whole different story! I couldn't reach the pedals and see over the dash at the same time. My cousin became my eyes. We would climb the hill and she would tell me if cars were coming. "Cars!" I would stomp the break pedal, the car would die, and we would roll backwards. Now, she becomes the traffic director. Hanging out the window, she is making hand signals to *get back* and *go around* to the cars on the hill behind us. After a half dozen tries, the coast was clear. So much for just parking it in the same place, and no one would ever know! All of those Police Cars were taking up the parking spaces. I'm thinking, "Where is the Police, when you need them? Are you telling me that they never heard or seen my brothers car across the street, from half a block away? We might have been killed!" Go ahead and ask me if I believe in Guardian Angels. I know they exist. I must have had a herd of them, working overtime, through my lifetime.

Adolescence was uneventful. I was the Tomboy, playing baseball, basketball, and football. Since the boys outnumbered the girls ten to one, if we wanted to play, we would have to play with the guys… we didn't have enough girls to make a team of anything. At sixteen, my Mother gave me a talk about becoming a lady. I should probably forget the rough and tumble games, and grow up. Well, the soft leather Indian Moccasins' were all the rage. It wasn't long after we had the "talk," that I kicked a field goal… which, I suspect, broke my middle toe. I would limp along all day at school, but as soon as I was close enough to the house to be seen, I would walk straight to my room and have a silent scream. I suffered for my disobedience. I couldn't disappoint my Mom. I was convinced that it was time to grow-up. I got a job. That pretty well kept me out of trouble.

The Young Lady would go on to work for the Government in Washington, DC. What an exciting time this was. I met people from all over the United States. It was a study in sociology; learning the lives and cultures of many people. This was a great opportunity for me. I had always loved nature and human nature. Washington was a city of great concerts, plays, restaurants, dancing, and clubs. It was a great jumping-off spot, to visit other places, also. We lived close to Rock Creek Park. This is one of the greatest places there is anywhere, to get-away-from-it-all. It is so calming and relaxing. A stroll through Rock Creek helped you *slow down and smell the roses*. What a wonderful time in my life, this was! I loved my job and loved my life. The only drawback? I sustained a "Southern Brogue," which is with me to this day! Missouri won't claim it, and Florida doesn't claim it. I was a girl without a Country, until I married a Texan. The Texans knew right away, that I was speaking correctly; even though I had never been West. (A real blessing is the fact that, to me, I sound just like everyone else.)

The Young Woman moved to Miami, married and had her children. I am thankful that I retain these memories. The first child was a picture of what his father would look like, when his father grows old. So healthy looking, he looked as if he came with a tan. (Perhaps a perk of being born in Miami Beach.) Everyone commented on *the baby with a tan.* Then came the second baby boy. Once again, making history upon his arrival, the second son was pink-skinned with platinum blond hair. He was *the only blond baby* in a nursery, that was a sea of brunettes. Can I say, they have always stood out in a crowd? A mother is allowed to boast. I'm glad I have my memories of these two exciting lives. I can't imagine being robbed of that! I am so lucky.

Of the many family vacations, one stands out among the rest. I call it "Gods Guided Tour." We drove through the West-Northwest. The sights were breath-taking. There was rain on the Painted Desert; which made all of the colors stand out. We arrived at the rim of the Grand Canyon, greeted by a double rainbow. For two little boys from Florida, the four inches of snow in Yellowstone, made for a great Fourth of July. (We had to drive with their little snowman on the hood of the car, till it melted.) They got to watch gunfights of the Old West, ate supper in a Teepee, watched the sunrise and the reflection in the lake, of the Grand Tetons. There were fields of wild flowers for as far as the eyes could see. The boys had fun picking special bouquets, just for me. I think that the reason this was such a great vacation, is that it came along before the boys would find interest in their own summer camps. It had been a memorable family occasion. Nothing quite that spectacular since.

The boys spent quite a few summers, visiting their cousins in Texas. Sure, I was aghast, when I learned that the children had bought that old Metropolitan Nash. Then, these kids learned to drive a car, all between the ages of 7 and 12. I had to trust the wisdom of their Uncle Tom. I was assured everything was safe; they only drove on a lonely road in the cemetery, so they couldn't hurt anyone. (Of course, their Uncle Tom was a lot like me: why bother someone with an impending disaster, when there may not be a disaster. I appreciate that, I think. Much like the other near disasters, I never knew about!) They were so happy and excited! "This was the best summer of our life!," they exclaimed. "What a great vacation!" (Yeah, sure!) I wonder if my boys knew how lucky they were? They will, now. I learned to drive when I was fourteen. My brother would tell me to take the old Chevy Coupe out on the Bay Road and practice. I would go out by myself and practice on those *Gravel Roads*; which was just a road full of large, loose rocks (the size of bowling balls). As I recall, it was more like skating, than driving! If I survived that, what's a cemetery? Of course, I would always remind myself of Route 66, also. Anything the boys did, seemed mild, compared to me; from their Go-Kart "pacer" to the Roadrunner "racer." Just in case, I've had an active prayer life.

How many people can say they enjoy their work? How many are able to help their fellow man, in such a pivotal way? Nurses are fortunate, that way. We relieve pain, perceived pain, or psychological pain. In all ways, we can give comfort; make their lives better or their passing easier. I am so blessed, and I know it. There are many fond memories of my patients. (Of course, the Nursing Class Grad Party, was quite memorable, too. Not to mention our State Boards. We would arrive at our motel the evening before our test, so we would be rested, bright-eyed and bushy-tailed for the early morning start of the tests. There were a few of us who didn't believe in last minute study; either you know it or you don't. We were the ones in the pool, most of the night! Maybe that is why our scores were so high; we were too sleepy to be *up-tight.* Just bring on the next test, so we can finish and get out of here.)

Scuba Diving and Underwater Photography were a challenge. We enjoyed sharing our pictures with friends who were afraid of the water, but were amazed at the beautiful creatures and scenery of the underwater world. The videos gave them the feeling of being there. Now, that is real relaxation! It is like the return to the amnion. You haven't a care in the world. It is so calming, floating around with the sea life, that you become a part of them. I find solace in the underwater world. The fish can sense that you mean them no harm, and so, are attracted to you. (Not unlike the people we meet.) How does one explain the fish that will follow you along your dive, like a puppy; stop and look under a ledge, when you stop and look under a ledge; follow you back to the boat and watch you depart the water? At times like that, it makes you realize, perhaps all life is smarter than we think them to be. Once you understand what miracles lie beneath the surface, you want to make an effort to preserve and protect them. Their future, is our future.

Is your glass half-full or half-empty? First, get yourself a positive attitude. It's not unusual, to be sitting around a table in some restaurant and hear similar conversations: I pass around a picture of some fish following me on my Dive. One girl will say, "Oh, I could never scuba dive. I have claustrophobia and I'm afraid of water. I don't even know how to swim. I'd drown." The other girl says, "I'd like to try Scuba one day. It looks like fun!" The first girl doesn't even have a glass half-empty; it is completely empty. For the second girl, her glass is still half-empty. "But wait, you say. She seems willing to learn something new." For her "*one day*" I'd say, "What are you doing tomorrow?" Like steel, good intentions erode with time. With a positive attitude, you might say, "I'm going to learn to fly. I love being in small planes." Even knowing that I don't have a spare penny to my name, I knew that I would become a pilot. It is the confidence and the determination that gets you where you want to go. Go on. I challenge you to make your glass half-full, and push for the topping. The best may be yet to come!

I've touched on many textures in my life: How can one explain the thrill of parasailing? It was something I saw, and needed to experience. The quiet was amazing. No sound of the wind, as in soaring. The fact that sounds rise, was fascinating. I could sail over someone down below and hear their most intimate whispers. I must remember that, when one sails by me. But then, Soaring makes you feel so free. You follow the paths of the birds; almost a holy experience for anyone, especially for the part of me that is American Indian. For a while, you let the air currents take control; just sit back and feel the floating. It reminds me of those times we dream of flying. (Personally, I like that feeling of weightlessness!)

Who would know that I could take Ground School for my elective in college? With the daily swimming and scuba diving, I wouldn't need more physical activity. With ground school out of the way, I would just have to wait until I could afford the flying lessons. So now I had finished Nursing School and gotten a job. Still, not a lot of money, feeding two teens with hollow legs; and not a lot of extra time. (When I became a Nurse, the first husband had moved-on, once he found that I could handle things on-my-own. As so often happens, the wives are there to do the bidding, of that adult spouse, who never grew up.) I promised myself I would never get into a situation like that again. Who needs an extra child to take care of? I don't care if I never date again! I'm a fun-loving person, so maybe when the kids are through college. Who knows? Right now, there is still kids to keep up with: homework, plays and concerts to attend, school outings, PTA's, and fit in as much listening and love as possible. Our greatest experiences still come from children. Is there more innocence or honesty anywhere? We enjoy the wisdom of our elders, also; if we are humble enough. Nurses and Teachers teach. May we always be curious and humble enough to learn from those we teach. Listen intently. The whole world has something to say, but few are listening.

About three years later, I met my Husband-to-be. Talking to his parents at Church, I noticed his father was wearing "wings" in his lapel. I told them that I was going to become a pilot, too. I'd already finished my ground school. They said that they would arrange for a flight in their small airplane, for that afternoon, if I liked. "That would be great!" Their son would be happy to take me for a flight. He'll give me a call. (I don't know. I'm not into blind dates, but how do you turn down a guy from Church?) He was so interesting and knowledgeable. (A bit of a show-off with the loop de loops. I promised to paint his instrument panel with vomit, if he didn't stop.) The plain flying in the plane was great. Now, we could just talk about likes and dislikes. I think that is why our marriage is so successful; nothing was left unsaid. I learned that he had always wanted to learn to Scuba Dive and never found time. He thought it interesting that I hoped to become a pilot, one day. But wait! He has an airplane I can use. He would need someone to *turn-the-oil-over* while he is taking his Scuba Lessons. (Am I lucky, or what?)

We chose healthful hobbies, to challenge our bodies and minds. Talk about "getting-away-from-it-all," Flying was the hobby of choice. Some of the closer Diving Trips did not depend on airline schedules; we could come and go, as we pleased. That was nice. We could also fly out to a small airport for dinner, to go shopping, hiking, sight-seeing, or just picnic. Then too, you could always visit friends or the kids at school. Still, you may prefer to just enjoy the scenery in flight; akin to doing nothing at all. It's a great hobby to help you relax, after a busy week at work.

The parasailing had this curious sole wondering about that time I had an out-of-body experience, from an allergic reaction to Tetracycline. I could never figure out how I was above the city, but could see everything going on. My eyes are in my head, and my head is in the car, so how do I see these things? (I had never been in a small plane before, in the early 60's.) When I started taking flying lessons, I realized that *my seeing* had been from about 1000 feet in the air. An interesting experience, but once was enough. I like being in control of myself, but this did give added dimension to my questions. Sure, I will always have questions. I guess that keeps life interesting.

We all learned to Scuba Dive and spent a few vacations in Cayman before the boys found other interest (School, Girls, Work, Girls, College, Girls, etc.) It was enjoyable, for the family to relax and play together in Cayman. (Where there just happened to be girls.) A study in Nature and Human Nature, again. I loved it! A visit or phone call from either of these two "boys," still brings indescribable joy. They have grown into admirable gentlemen.

There are so many textures to our lives. Where do they come from? Usually, it is not by chance or coincidence. It is by time planned and scheduled. Grab the fun and run! Learn to Live Each Day to the Fullest! Time is precious. We should grab 10% of our time for ourselves; to do just what we want to do. That is only a couple of hours a day. We can all find two hours of relaxing enjoyment each day. You will, however, have to plan ahead for that Vacation Time. Remember 10% of your time is equal to 36 days of vacation every year. It need not be all at once; plan short exploring trips on long weekends. See the relatives on the Holidays.

It works for us. We've seen so much and learned so many new things, from our short adventure trips.

My Husband and I arrange our schedules around the Afternoon Shifts at work. Mornings are then open to adventure. We also plan two longer vacation trips a year; one in the Spring and one in the Fall. These are usually scuba diving trips out of the Country. Plan them all year. It gives you something to look forward to, as the excitement grows. This is my schedule: Fit-in that two hours for yourself, to do just what you want to do. Don't let anything interfere with your schedule. For that 2 hrs., I belong to Me, to do as I please. Then, when I go to work, I belong to and am dedicated to my job. After work, I belong to my Husband. He is my best friend and we are as one. Plan Your Happiness!

Don't become a Workaholic! When your shift is done and you leave work, leave the job behind! Have some fun and talk "happy talk."

* * * * * * *

With all of the textures I have touched, my life is full. In the scheme of things, these past ten years have been, but one small chapter, in the story of my life.

Study the Textures you have sown.
Dig Deep.
You'll be surprised and in awe,
by the memories you seek.
All of those textures you have known;
you cannot let them sleep
All of the ways that you have grown;
Are Memories to share and keep.

* * * * * * *

One would think that I would have recognized my out-of-body experience with the Near-Electrocution much earlier, having experienced it before with the antibiotics; but, with the brain injury, nothing came together. Wouldn't I wonder how I maintained such an indelible movie of the whole thing? Not a hint, for years. Then, I realized it would always be there; it was burned on my mind, like my own *"Last Picture Show!"* I'm guessing, this had been the very

LAST MEMORY OF MY PAST LIFE.

* * * * * * *

CHAPTER 17

IN THE SCHEME OF THINGS

IN THE SCHEME OF THINGS,

Yes, this had been, but one small chapter in the story of my life. Even so, I can share the insight with others, who may see themselves in my plight. No matter what journey we encounter or what challenges we face, each really is just a small part of the whole. When we think of all of the wonderful things we've done, we are thankful for all experiences. We have the ability to cull them, and choose which ones will become significant. So, is the cup half full, or half empty?

I'm sorry I can no longer fly my plane, but I am grateful for the journey. I loved every minute of it. When I think of this, I am grateful that I had retained my past memories. I really was quite fortunate, you know. Gliding along some coral reef, taking pictures of a menagerie of the Undersea World, was exquisite. But, there is nothing that can compare with the joy of birth and watching my little ones grow-up. I have so many fond memories! I especially enjoyed their laughter, through the years:

How does anyone explain the way a child can defy gravity, with their building blocks. (Go ahead and get the camera for proof of this architectural wonder. It will come tumbling down, the minute you lift the camera.) Don't tell me that children do not have guardian angels. I've seen too much. How might I explain a two-year-old, sitting in the middle of the bathroom floor; quiet for a while, and then letting out a hilarious laugh. I was vacuuming, and *of course* he was taking a nap. Sure! Imagine my surprise when I found him with my giant box of tampons, shooting them all over the room. He can't have figured that out for himself! He learned to walk early, and was in to everything. During that time, we lived in Texas. In all of his first pictures, he was dressed in cowboy garb. (Maybe that is why he thinks he is a Texan.) As he grew older, he introduced us to his *imaginary friend*, Drewer. (We might as well blame Drewer for all of the past mysterious happenings.) When *The First Born* was old enough to talk, he blamed everything on Drewer. The first child is always the *talker*. I don't know why, but we always push that first child to talk. (Maybe, we were bored with so much peace and quiet.) He had acquired a huge vocabulary by age three, and he never stopped. This put him ahead of the rest of his class. Boredom is never good.

He had the usual paper route, and collection day was always a long drawn-out affair. He could talk a snake out of its' rattlers. In Boy Scouts, he won the Soapbox Derby. It would be at the awards ceremony, when he had the *open fly*. (Media Coverage!) Then, came Sea Cadets. It amazed me, how he required his charges to bounce a quarter on their beds, while his bed at home, did well to even have the linens on it. (Though, I must admit, I enjoyed the fellow cadets asking who his girlfriend was. The blonde who picked him up from Sea Cadets, in that shinny red car.) It was "The Sea Cadets on Parade," for St. Patrick's Day.

"Tex" had his new schoolmates convinced he was from Texas; even the accent seemed genuine. This was a great way to start the school year, at his new Christian School! I don't know why we paid for bus service; he was always staying after school. We would have to make a special trip, to retrieve him. Either the school was too conservative or he was too liberal thinking. His love for debating and intellectual reasoning, had no place in this school! Far from the theory of public school: not to inhibit their growth.

His Halloween costumes were always gross. The teenager answered the phone, while rinsing his dishes.... "Sure, I'll get you that number. Let me go back into my room and get my directory." The water spilling over the sink, would flow through the wall, through the closet, and across the master bedroom's carpeting; so I'm told, eventually. There would be the Chorus trips to Disney World, the Dance Champ, and Auto Racer. He worked as a Stockroom Clerk, became a Bank Cashier, Dog Track Cashier, Jai Alai Cashier, worked in a Funeral Home doing "pick-up & delivery," was a Waiter, and Bartender. His most difficult job was, deciding on the right Majors for college. It's rough attending the best "Party School" in the Country. You will be pleased to know that he used most of his various Majors. (Still, the Mixology Course taken, while working at college, guaranteed invites to all parties.) The Finance Degree sent him on to Corporate Banking Loans and Travel. His real interest became Sales Representative, where he was in contact with more people. He has a genuine interest in helping others. Volunteer work helps, in that department. He's a fine young man. First, to thine own self, be true.

Along came my second son, five years later. What a joy! Two individual personalities, as different as night and day. I would not want it any other way. I don't remember this younger child ever having taken a nap. He might have gotten tired, but naps were not for him. He was still in a pleasant mood, no matter how tired he was. How could you argue with that? At night, he would have those long talks with his Grandfather; then, would be too tired to eat his breakfast. Once, he came home with his blond hair matted with blood. Kenneth had thrown a concrete block off of the roof, and hit him on the head. (Who says that cartoons are harmless?! Young and impressionable children, should never see cartoons!) Billy and he baked cupcakes, on top of the stove, as a surprise for me. (Oh, I was surprised!) Billy had a wild croquet swing. Of course, all I heard was, " Billy knocked my eye out," as *My Baby* cupped his hand over his eye socket. Oh, no! I had seen the results of an eye being knocked out before. Just home from a long shift in the ER, I was relieved to find the eye intact. (Couldn't he have put a flat hand over it?) These two were clowns in the St. Patrick's Day Parade. They were pretty funny, most of the time, anyway. Little Barnee Beagle, bluffed as the dominant dog. Maybe that is why Sheepdog Ralff, learned he could climb trees. The boys thought that great fun!

Hanging clothes on his birthday?! (Well, I had to frost his cake!) This convinced him it was true, when his brother teased, "You're adopted, anyway!" I wonder how that plays out with the Mailman? Wasn't he supposed to be the real father? At least, that's what we had heard. (Life is not always easy, for a Sunday School Teacher; nor, for the Mailman, for that matter.) The youngest is always teased mercilessly. (Would you believe, these two brothers are the Best-of-Friends today?! I guess there is hope for everyone.)

Their yearly trip to Texas, let a child be a child. They enjoyed their cousins. One Summer, they learned the responsibility of earning money to buy a car, by *hoeing cotton.* They all worked together and bought this little Metropolitan Nash, and each one learned to drive... at much too young an age! Well, that's alright! He was a good kid, and everyone survived. (There is always my driving history!)

I worked hard, but tried to repaint the woodwork every two to three years. I did get the baseboards scrubbed and sanded before going on vacation. He decided to paint them for me, as a nice surprise. I understand he spilled a paint tray-full of white paint, on the blue carpeting; but would we ever know?

He saved his *open fly* for the High School Play. Boys are very reliable about one thing; they will embarrass you with an open fly. We just never know when. (I think it usually occurs, during expected High Media Coverage!)

He was another Dance Champ and attended Summer Camps. Sharks in the pool? There appeared to be. Our pool was not twelve feet deep, so we had no diving board. That seemed pretty safe! Who would have guessed, that they were running across the roof and clearing a six-foot patio, to dive into the pool. Do insurance adjusters get that same uncomfortable feeling on the back of their necks, as we parents had? We may not have had Crime Watch in those days, but I sure am thankful for the **Neighbors Watching**. Those boys never got by with much. (Sure, it takes a village to raise a child.)

This son, preferred *Dracula* or *The Grapes of Wrath,* for Halloween. Of course, there were the Disney Trips with the High School Chorus. We can't forget his Roadrunner Car. For Graduation, my in-laws gave him a sexy *Photo Shoot.* He would become a Grocery Checker, Shoe Salesman, worked for a TV Channel (during college), and then on to work for a Real Estate Data company. Another fine gentleman, ready to help his community. He works hard, but then, he plays hard: White-Water racing, Skiing vacation, Rain Forest ventures, and Plateau censures.

Flying kites, riding bikes, Go-Kart runs, Metropolitan fun, Hugs & Kisses, Long Distance misses. There were Peanut Vendors and 757 Rocket-Senders. Dogs and little boys, Birthday Cakes and Christmas toys. Graduations and Family Vacations. *Assembly line* matching shirts. The fun of "Old Fashion Day" at Church. The Wedding Cake and the bathroom mistake. Both boys had such interesting friends and dates. It was a very happy time. I am so glad that I still have these memories of mine.

* * * * * * *

Why is it so difficult for Mothers to let their children go, in every stage of their growing-up; kindergarten, first grade, summer camp, sixth grade, ninth grade, high school, graduations, college, moving away, etc.? Because we were there to enjoy all of those little things that only a Mother secretly remembers: How they giggled together, strategic arguing, playing tricks on everyone, singing together songs of struggles and victories, reliving the days happenings, favorite books, stories, and board games, etc. All, great memories!

Though, we spoke of the *cup-cake caper*, the way *too-long phone conversations, white paint on blue carpeting*, and *open flies*; I would direct your attention to some other valuable enlightening times: He came home with a beautiful bouquet of roses, from some unsuspecting neighbor along the way, because he knew how much his Mother loved flowers. (How do you ask, "Where did you get those? They are beautiful, but they don't belong to us. Someone planted them to share with the whole world, not just you and me. We must take them back and apologize.") No one says it is going to be easy, being a parent! But, it sure is entertaining. I stopped by the drugstore to pick-up a prescription. When we returned to the car, I noticed that my four-year-old was playing with a little car. Here we go again, "Where did you get that?" (In there, as he pointed to the drugstore.) "That man sells those toys so he can feed his kids. They are not free. You have to pay for them. You will have to take it back to the manager and tell him you're sorry and promise never to do that again." (The manager wanted to give it to him for his honesty, but we refused, saying we had toys at home.) See, you may have learned something new today: You may have gotten past the *terrible twos*, but watch out for the *three and four-year old thieves*. Come to think of it, *pre-twos* could be quite a challenge, also. It was so cute, when he learned to pull-up on the tripod of my easel; his thorough finger painting ended my desire to do oil paintings, again. It was obvious, I would need to focus my attention on the young *sleep-walkers*; you know, the ones who are supposed to be taking naps. (Perhaps, when they finish college.) The crepe dress I designed and seed-smocked until I was half blind, would need ingenuity to repair the half-circle cut through the sleeve in the back. (Cut an identical design on the other side and sew both with a thin seam; it just looked like a shoulder tuck.) We survived: the Alvin records, and Benjamin Brownie books. Home-made books of their dog "Bar-Nee Beagle" and the "Hospital Visit." Kindergarten craft gifts (some of which I still possess.) Swimming lessons. The driving lessons. My list goes on, but many you have read about in this book. It's a wonderful life.

I just keep telling myself over and over again, just how fortunate I am to, at least, have my memories of the past.

IF ALL OF MY PAST MEMORIES

WERE NOT GOOD ENOUGH FOR ME,

THEN, JUST HOW UNGRATEFUL WOULD I BE?

* * * * * * *

PS: Just when you think that parenting is a thankless job, a specific "Thank You" comes along: It would be several years later, when my son said he wanted to thank me. (I'm wondering, "What for?") He always remembered the matchbox car, he took from the drugstore. When other pre-teens and teens were swiping stuff or laughing about five-finger-discounts, he was never ever tempted to steal anything and he wanted to thank me for that early lesson! Yes, tears well-up in my eyes, to think I made a difference. As parents, we can only try; but really, their character makes the difference. And, my other son is aware of my love for flowers, but he has always bought them for me, since that first bouquet. Sure, the smell of Cotton Candy will always remind me of the cupcakes, cooked on top of the stove. (It's the thought that counts! He made them just for me, because I was so busy studying for a college exam, I never took a break.) Many times, they just wanted to do something nice for me; then I had to *rain-on-their-parade*, by preaching justice. Every instance I look back at, brings a smile. I'm sure, my boys see these instances quite differently than I. They probably thought me to be disappointed and displeased with them. I hope not. These were just little lessons to be taught. Always let them know you love them. I will forever see them as sweet little angels, just needing guidance. They are my pride and joy!

All agree that we were right to insist on wearing seatbelts, long before it was compulsory; this has paid-off for all of us.

No Smoking was an intelligent choice for both boys. When given the facts, your children can make logical decisions on their own. Are you too, still thinking that parenting is a thankless job? Just look at the fine children who grew-up to be fabulous adults! (Listen closely, you just may hear them repeating the wisdom you expounded to them.) I'm thankful for the opportunity to teach life's lessons; knowing that most lessons are taught, by setting an example.

OH, YES

CHILDREN WILL BE, WHAT CHILDREN SEE !

How fortunate I've been!

What a great family and a great life!

%%%%%%%%%%

LIFE

Our life is a collage of memories and dreams.
Some are pursued, while some are unseen.

As a baby, we grow into the child,
adolescent, teen; and all the while,

chasing new adventures and textures to taste.
Not for a moment of time to waste.

Life is not always smooth silk, I've found;
There is a lot of rough tweed, going around.

So, whether the textures are smooth or coarse,
Not tasting at all, would have been worse.

%%%%%%%%%%

THE CAN-DO GIRL.

As for me, **THE "CAN-DO GIRL"** has found a lot of things she CAN DO. It's **good**, that I can put my blouse on over my head, and it comes out right… no more tags in the front! It's **very good** that I can laugh at myself, when the wrong words roll off my tongue, or no words come at all. My assimilation comes easier and, perhaps, a bit faster. (O.K. reading a newspaper still takes forever; it is still small print, on which the lines run together. FRUSTRATION!) The wit has returned, but not as quick. It's still good for a chuckle. I can still give away a smile and conversation to strangers. This is a great joy! I can fix and assemble a meal, in proper order, as long as I don't get a lot of feed-back from some talker, asking questions that have nothing to do with what I am currently doing. (The old *changing mode* game.) I can do the routine chores around the house; laundry, cleaning, gardening, etc. With the help of my husband, I can keep up with the family calendar. You know, the dental appointments, club meetings, birthdays, visitors coming and going, etc. (We were once a lost civilization.) By zooming-in on the things you can do, it will encourage you to keep on trying. You never know what is in store for tomorrow. This one thing I know! **Expect great things of GOD, to beget great things from GOD!** Then, put feet under your prayers. You see, NOW, I CAN DO a lot more than before!

I'm okay with **ME**!

PSSSSSSSSSSSSSSSST !!!

Some have suggested that my book would be a good pre-requisite for the Pre-med and the Pre-law students. See how many medical mistakes were made. See how many civil liberty abuses you could find. There is enough blame for everyone. But, the truth of the matter remains, my case is not so unusual. There are many with disabilities, who are being denied rightful compensation, for injuries received on the job. So, is Workers Comp just another farce; giving us some sort of false comfort, knowing that our tax dollars are helping the people who can not help themselves? Rarely, would you find an honest broker, who would truly look out for the interest of the disabled. It is not easy to jump through the hoops and red tape, put before us, when many of us have no advocate to file our case. We are treated as if there are no disabilities to contend with; perhaps to weed-out the frauds. However, these papers are for someone capable of comprehending the instructions, deciphering the questions, assimilating the answer, while trying to construct the appropriate sentence; certainly not for a person with a new brain injury. I'm speaking from experience. Like I've said, the disadvantaged are not represented, but rather, taken advantage of. I don't care how many laws we have on the books; if they are not enforced, how effective can they be? Black Lung, Chemical Exposure, Carpal Tunnel, etc., are just a few examples. With Carpal Tunnel Syndrome, the Companies complain that it would cost too much, if they tried to take care of all of the people affected. (Maybe they should try to prevent it!) And, don't we wish that judges could walk in the shoes of the disabled, for just one day? Like many HMO's, it is all about the bottom line! If companies can't afford to pay for these injuries, how about preventative measures? It would be much cheaper, in the long run. Now, how do we justify, or correct, the deficits? By education. We will go, only as far, as we are willing to put forth the effort. Leaders must take the initiative, and

SEE TO IT, THAT OUR DISABLED,
DO NOT BECOME OUR DISADVANTAGED!

Let's clean up our messes.

WHAT DO YOU THINK?

?

POSTSCRIPT:

I'm doing great! Whether it is from improvement or acceptance, is unimportant. Learning to love yourself again is very important; in order to get-on with your life, and to enjoy it to the best of your ability. Try to see the fun and beauty in every new experience. Then, pass-it-on to others you meet. When we take the time to look back at our life, we find so many wonderful memories. You really appreciate those great boys, a loving husband, and the remarkable family and friends. Even some of the strangers we've met along the way, gave us precious memories to cling-to. Sure, my most recent meetings will have been forgotten, but the beauty remains that strangers are still like ourselves; they are just passing through and are going to do the best they can, while on their journey. We love the generous hearts, the friendly greetings, and the helping hands we've met along the way.

What are we doing for recreation; for passing the time:

In retirement, there is no time limit, so time seems limitless. Think again! I don't know how we ever got things done, while working and running a household. Even in my FOG in California, I was having great fun; I just wouldn't remember it. It seemed to me, that all I was doing was skating as fast as I could, to catch-up with life; or was I just trying to catch reality? With my Short-Term Memory, I won't remember any of our California Adventures; good or bad. (My rampant mistreatment could leave a bad taste in my mouth, from our California Encounters. Hey, Wait! We Cockeyed Optimist will never permit negativity to rule our lives. I was just as glad to leave the whole thing buried and forgotten in some old mine shaft; a time-capsule left in the past.) Sure, I would have been happy, forgetting the whole experience; but too much of my life is missing. I need to recapture the life, outside of that Medical Progress Diary.

I'm sure I must have had some good times, but I can't remember. Then, my husband would open a whole new world for me. He would remind me of our good times. I'm grateful that my husband took his video camera, on each new adventure. The videos of our good times and good friends, shines a better light on our Adventures, ***over-shadowing our Misadventures***.

Nothing worth watching on TV? Who cares? We just pull out a CD of our past adventures and relive them. So, I am just now enjoying the scenic views, parks, and other attractions we visited, while there. The neighbors, block parties, the visits from friends and relatives with sight-seeing tours; all recorded for my enjoyment. Might I suggest that you start your own Personal Video Collections? It's a delight! Enjoy those good times, every chance you get.

While I enjoy socializing, I think I'm most comfortable on a hiking trail. I don't have to worry about *changing modes,* fixing meals at a certain time, being home by a certain time, or turning out a clever conversation. There are always things of interest to see, scenery for taking photos, people to meet… just more CD's to make of all of my present fun! I'll keep that media growing! I sure have fun reliving these things. That doesn't mean, however, I will settle for this. There is still so many things to do and so many things to see. They are all just waiting for you and for me.

Socializing opportunities are boundless. A trip to the Mall, is still a lot of fun. I enjoy the beauty of Human Nature. You are in contact with people of all ages, and can find out about the latest fads. (I'm still not so sure about the latest language!) Remember, that Outing keeps you in touch with the rest of the world; at least, the World as we know it.

Take a friend shopping. We may not buy a thing, but that wasn't what it was all about anyway. It was just some time alone, to do some *girl talk* and *goof-off;* to let our hair down. Movies are great social trips, also. While coming in or leaving, in those long lines, you have a chance to practice your *small talk.* Bashful? Get out there anyway. You will get used to it. It will become fun & something to look forward to. So many little things bring much joy; and don't cost a thing, but time.

Is it difficult finding a volunteer program? Just find something that fits your abilities. I can now, research subjects on the computer for others. (I won't have to worry about using an inappropriate word; or the loss for words. It is quite satisfying to be able to help.) Volunteering gives you an increased sense of self-worth. That can't be bad!

Whatever you choose to do, get out there. Some of the greatest ideas come from the disabled. Is there something that bugs you about your wheelchair? Think of a solution! What could you use, to make things better? Maybe your blanket drags in the wheels. Find a large rubber band or a large Velcro strap to keep it gathered on you lap. I don't know; that may help. I'll bet you have better ideas. Don't waste your time letting others find your solutions, when you can think of them yourself. It makes you feel good about you!

I can plant a flower bed; however, my brown thumb is still brown. I buy plants that are already in bloom, and the place looks great (until they die and I have to plant others.) Oh well, the seasons change anyway, and you will need a color change.

I am still working on my future adventures and the video camera stands at "ready." Meanwhile, let me encourage you to write about your life and make videos of special occasions. Looking at the videos and reading the stories, are real joys.

You may just find that things you are doing now, may remind you later, of the great progress you've made. Good Luck!

I know I am lucky. My memories are of times past, but they bring back great memories... Things I can never do again, but things to remember, way back when.

TEXTURES OF MY LIFE.

Taking my little hand in hers,
as we walked along,
My Mother would sing to me,
many wonderful songs.

The curious child wondered why
we couldn't always be "Together."
It was not in Gods plan.
I couldn't marry Daddy either.

Someday, I would have children,
when I was all grown;
then, my children would need a Daddy,
who was all their own.

This little girl didn't understand
that her family was poor;
and was always proud of those pretty
flour-sack dresses that she wore.

My Daddy ate the food I cooked,
in my little girls pans.
Can you imagine the bravery,
of this fabulous man?

I was my big brother's pesky
tag-along *aggravator*.
Till I became my little brothers
agitating troublemaker.

Like the people in the grocery store,
eating green-colored grapes;
we ate our Concords green
and had such stomach aches.

Daddy read us stories,
when we were still quite young.
Then, we would have to act them out,
each and every one.

We had to grow up, in the same County,
as did Tom and Huck;
I would wish for every child,
the same adventurous luck.

Building rafts, roaming hills, exploring caves,
sliding down red clay mounds and
climbing shale cliffs, along the way
(they call it *rock-climbing*, today.)

Wading the creek in Summer,
looking for crawdads; finding snakes.
The creek seemed safer in Winter,
when we'd play "Silver Skates."

My Mother played "Hide and Seek,"
though she would often win.
Or, did we let her catch us,
'cause she hugged us to her chin?

Daddy taught us astrology,
all gathered under the stars.
Perhaps, this is why I'm still awed,
by a shooting star.

We loved that big old swing,
tied high in the Hickory Tree.
Together, the seat was wide enough,
for <u>both</u> Ellen and me.

We got to play with my tea set,
but "hands through the fence";
though, we never quite understood
our dubious offense.

We were just two little girls
giggling with glee,
you could never ever
take away that memory!

My Dad's baseball games were always fun,
for family and fans.
If his team won, he entertained,
by walking on his hands.

We kids spent time in the corners,
when being "noisy clowns."
My (smart aleck) big brother, served <u>one time</u>,
turned up-side-down.

I remember the yellow Butterflies
upon the purple Thistle,
and chasing all those Fireflies,
until the bedtime whistle.

There was a garden of colorful Hollyhocks,
some high and some low.
Be careful, when smelling them.
A Bumblebee might sting your nose.

Our own "Sleepy Hollow" filled we young ones
with terrible fright.
But then came knowledge; and with age,
it would give us that very same might.

Hot summer nights, we slept out in the yard;
on pallets upon the grass.
To get us quiet to go to sleep,
"The Headless Horseman" passed.

How did my Dad make that noise of hooves?
or, was *the real thing*, passing our place?
We covered our heads and went to sleep;
To save <u>our heads</u>, just in case.

It was always a thrill, riding in Grandma's
classy rumble-seat car.
In our *convertible*, we girls became
glamorous Hollywood Stars.

The Outhouse was a common joke,
for all of our friends and kin.
But, I never found it amusing,
come the Winter wind.

Were there "Crop Circles"
out in those alfalfa fields?
Everyone could tell you, Certainly,
"They were really real!"

The Fourth of July was for a
Family Gathering; a party, out our way.
Just outside of the City Limits,
made all of our fireworks okay.

The neighborhood Outdoor Movies,
were fascinating treats.
My uncle showed the latest movies,
to distract from the summer heat.

The scary Seance with mystical flair,
caused panic, when spiders fell out of the air.

It was "Sheena of the Jungle" and "Me, Jane,"
traversing *our jungle* on the grapevine swings.

We were hiding high in our tree-house retreats,
spying on the boys, those "neighborhood creeps."
Biking those hot summers, when just on a whim,
cooling off in water holes, though we couldn't swim.

THE ADOLESCENT RITE OF PASSAGE:

Trying to smoke weed, way back when
"weed" meant simply a milkweed stem.

At age twelve, we got our kicks,
driving the car, on Route 66.

My brother taught me how to drive,
around the age of fourteen.
Probably, he saved my life;
if you know what I mean.

We won many dance contests,
for prizes we couldn't use;
A *fine cut-glass wine decanter*,
or a big old bottle of booze!

We have no fear, and very little sense,
during those years, we call adolescence.

* * * * * * *

It is a blessing, when your family life is so rich with love, you don't even know you are poor.

The family *board-games* with popcorn,
would turn into family *card games* and popcorn.

Some family traditions are worth carrying on.
A card game is easy inclusion, for most everyone.

From the High School Play to the Skip School Day,
Teenage years were so busy, it was a dizzying maze.

My first job was in the Hardware Department,
of the local department store.
It gave this very curious teen, many interesting
tools and gadgets to explore.

To receive the Biology grade, I did pass the snake,
(but with a fling.)
Hitting a cabinet in the back of the room;
did they ever find the poor thing?

Most of the girls were sophisticated, and
anxious to get-on-our-way.
While the boys were still testing beer;
with a *Devil May Care* display.

* * * * * * *

THOSE LATE TEENS AND EARLY TWENTIES.

I'm going to The Big City,
and I can hardly wait.
I had planned on this event,
since I was barely eight.

Living with six roommates,
made for a happy congregation.
We'd find so many things to do;
with so much imagination.

We enjoyed teaching Dance
to the Servicemen, at the YWCA.
(A bit of friendly charity,
after a long workday.)

It took a lot gumption
for the small-town girl, who was so shy.
As usual, I will challenge myself,
in everything I try.
I was voted the Best Dressed,
in our Department at work.
Still wearing my pretty flour-sack dresses,
didn't seem to hurt.

Perhaps this *Shy One* needed,
that vote of confidence.
No pretending, I would still be me,
and keep that innocence.

The dress stores in our hometown,
had sold 9's and 10's, in size.
In the City, I would find,
I really wore a size 5.

Some Servicemen took us to see,
our first ***Submarine Race***.
A roommate's brother and family friend,
sure helped us all save-face.

Sailing at Annapolis, the water was rough,
with a very cold spray.
I thought that we would freeze to death,
on that Autumn day.

From *Mickey Mantle* at the bat,
in my softball games;
we would all, then, go cool-off,
on the playground swings.

Living next door to a Georgetown
Paternity House, kept us all on guard.
Their Halloween punch was in a bathtub,
they got from an old junkyard.

They wouldn't need to clean the
gigantic bathtub ring, 'cause

the concoction they put in it,
would sanitize anything.

Had they really thought of us, as just
Some Dumb Blondes? Say it isn't so!
Giving a *Precious Ring* from a gum machine,
thinking we wouldn't know???

Spent New Year's Eve
in Times Square.
It was "Windy" in the City,
without a care.

Did the hula-hoop on the tabletop,
for St. Patrick's Day;
confident in the fact, "No one
is going to remember this, anyway!"

The local tonsillectomy, gave Medics
their very first thought;
I should never have Opium again!
No! No matter what.

The changing DC weather
left my *sinuses such a mess.*
The doctor told me to, "Move,
if you want any rest."

He suggested Arizona,
but that's just too dry.
I'm a Water Baby.
I need water to survive.

I had foiled a crazy abduction;
but, do I really need this pace?
I will seek a day-shift job,
in another place.

I'll go to Florida. Shirley lived there
and made it sound like fun.
Tropical Fruits and warm weather,
with lots of sand and sun.

Having so many roommates
from all over the USA,
left me with a *Southern Brogue*,
so my friends would say.

South Florida, a mixture of cultures;
just like it was in DC.
This meant, I would not stand-out.
I could just be me.

I loved the solitude of quiet, relaxing,
moonlit phosphorescent swims;
millions of shiny *pearls* would appear,
with each arm's gentle skim.

We *"lived-on-the-beach,"* daily;
via Greyhound Bus, for the fun!
Chasing the shade of a palm tree,
to stay out of the noon-day sun.

One house we rented, reminded me
of an old orange crate, circa '23,
with the glass chandelier reading 100 watts,
and 22 jalousies.

Cranking 22 jalousie windows,
seemed way beyond our powers.
Only *new-comers* would rent this place;
there are always afternoon thunder showers!

The suave dates, with Brazilian Businessmen,
had its noisy distractions.

The roommates stirred-up barking dogs,
by counting on garbage can traction.
(Never step on a cocked-lid top, to climb any direction.)

Though I hadn't driven since age fourteen,
(my brother taught me, from pity).
As "Girl Friday," I ***picked-up and delivered cars***;
all over this Big City.

Miami was such an exciting place.
It was one party after another.
Lifeguards galore and the usual Marines,
were all friends of each other.

We enjoyed those evening beach picnics,
with all of the food we made.
Cooling off in the *Ocean of Pearls*,
while "Moon Over Miami" played.

I'd have plenty of time for marriage;
I'll wait till I'm, at least, thirty-five.
But, with that big old Miami Moon,
how could you keep that dream alive?

Then, Daytona Beach was beautiful enough
for anyone's Honeymoon.
The wide white-sand beaches, caught
long shadows, in the afternoon.

ADULTHOOD:

Those teenage years, everyone would
remember as great fun;
but, how would we ever know?
We were always on-the-run.

When we settle into another era,
we think of things left undone.
The games lost, became more important,
than the ones you won.

If we are to learn Life's Lessons,
we must question everything.
Could I have played much better,
or just needed to play the game?

While you rein in the kid,
you allow them space to grow.
Making their own decisions early,
puts them *in-the-know.*

There were those who grew up
in *dysfunctional families*, as such.
Some parents didn't care enough; yet,
there were those who cared too much.

You teach the child what's right.
There is a happy medium, somewhere.
So, trusting the teen to make the right choice,
Shows them you really care.

With the transient family,
our childhood friends, gradually disappear.
Keeping in touch scarcely,
over their moves, miles, and years.

* * * * * * *

Yes, we married and had two sons,
which kept our lives exciting.
Filled with laughter along the way;
their smiles were so inviting.

Moving on into adulthood now,
became a much more serious plot.
Settling into a married life, makes you
grow-up, *"ready-or-not."*
The wonder of watching these two little boys,
growing up before your eyes.
There is nothing to bring more joy.
This, no parent could ever deny.

Millions of memories tucked in my heart.
How would they ever know?
Is it the proud way we look at them,
that tells them this is so?

When we visited Missouri,
the "Boys" took part in a Country Jam.
They enjoyed a family tradition,
with a guitar and banjo in their hands.

Why, they could become Stars
in the Western Band;
creating music, like our
Country/Western kin.

Summers with their cousins in Texas,
also, seemed like Heaven.
The youngest learned to drive a car,
when he was six or seven.

My two little boys grew into young men,
but, much too fast;
leaving their busy childhood dreams,
cradled in the past.

Wherever he went, *the first-born*
received his Birthday Cake,
Whether away at college
or in some distant State.

I made him a life-sized Teddy Bear,
before we moved away.

So, *my baby* could have a *big bear hug*,
any time of day.

See, we're proud they cut-the-apron-strings,
so confident and grown.
It's Moms that have ambivalence;
we'd like to keep them home.

Now, the *Boys* are grown and on their own;
their stories keep us spellbound.
We laugh about all of those things they did,
when we were not around.

The in-laws came to the rescue,
and we would never know.
Cleaning white paint from blue carpeting,
so it wouldn't show.

Then, there was the lifting of the carpeting
and large rented fans for drying.
A lot of work was needed, for <u>this</u> over-flow;
so everyone kept trying.

We enjoyed the Second Honeymoon,
and never noticed the difference.
They would all confess, and laugh about it,
in a safe (10 year) distance.

Sure, I married and had children; became
that stay-at-home Mom.
Then, went back to college, sharing books
with my oldest son.

I became **a Nurse**, along the way.
I had so much to give.
I enjoyed this fulfilling career.
It was **a *Mission* I could live**.

Learning to Scuba Dive, way back when,
Diving was the domain, of the Macho Man!

Went Parasailing in ’72.
When Parasailing was something new.

Took flying instructions. I just had to fly.
A whole other world, I needed to try.

Traveling the World, in these exciting times.
There are Oceans to see and Mountains to climb.

With Air Ambulance Rescues,
there were always exciting cases.
While meeting the needs of our patients,
we’ve seen many foreign places.

Sure, it’s easy to become spoiled
by South Florida’s water and sun.
Water temperatures were a warm welcome,
for all of your sporting fun.

Diving was so easy,
wherever you chose your ramp.
Whether Hollywood or Marathon,
or perhaps, Pennekamp.

The Bahamas were so close, yet so far;
lost to some *distant* cay.
The beauty and multi-hued waters,
let you step into that *Monet*.

Cayman called to everyone;
a whisper in the divers ear.
Come visit this Diving Mecca,
at least, every couple of years.

Bonaire would persuade you to try
the very same thing, if you possibly can.
A beautiful diving adventure awaits; again,
with people you understand.

How about the Yucatan?
We can't forget a Cozumel destination.
The easy-going lifestyle,
assures you a quiet, relaxing vacation.

Let's not forget the Virgins, which
enchant us, from *right next door.*
The British and the U.S. Virgins,
offer great sailing and fishing, galore.

So many little Caribbean Islands,
to explore and to choose from.
You will notice, they all have,
warm water and plenty of sun.

We loved the little towns,
with dirt roads and wooden paths.
The happy, easy-going people,
laugh and sing while doing their tasks.

There were no crowds to bother them.
There is this *Lovely Peace and Quiet*.
One could actually **listen to nature** and
see the stars at night.

The snorkeling (or scuba) was so easy,
from Maui's Black Rock Inn.
You can watch the fish feeding, and dry-off
on the sand; all, by sunset's end.

We've had a lot of fun, you see, but
not all vacations were totally trouble-free.

Now, they bring an uproarious laugh,
to my husband and me.....

How would you like to be
half-way around the world; so far from home?
The baggage handlers had broken the wheels off,
our **gigantic** roll-along!

Try maneuvering that, while looking for a hotel,
that didn't seem to exist.
Even the Police couldn't find the place.
What sort of a Scam was this?!

(Okay, so the Hotel had changed its' name,
but not yet changed the sign.
I guess we forgave the strange mix-up,
'cause we had such a great time!)

We found the Aussies were really
a breed of their own.
We loved these good-hearted people;
all *down-home* grown.

They have their priorities listed right;
guess what's number one?
(No. Work is way down on the list!)
First, is **having fun!!**

When we came to visit Australia and her
Great Barrier Reef,
we found the sights were so much more,
than even our wildest beliefs!

It was that *Once-in-a-Lifetime Vacation*,
to the World's Greatest Dive Spot!
But, my close-up attachment was lost.
I'd need to guess at every shot.

I would have to follow my "Trouble Shooting"
instructions, to-the-letter.
I'm here to tell you, that these pictures,
could not have come out better.

Still, any photo-diver will tell you,
the best ones get away.
After the last shot, the Dolphins jump,
and the Rays want to play.

I'm still enjoying their stories, though,
their brogue was worse than mine.
It's embarrassing to **laugh out-loud**,
after the rest of the crowd had waned.

We've found the Caribbean,
a very nice place to roam;
so many islands to choose from,
and yet, so close to home.

We had always liked to rent a car,
and seek our own special thrills.
Little did we know, that there were
Rebels in those hills!

The over-flight of Cuba, while innocent,
was not too wise.
We had the biggest "Mig Migraines,"
while over Cuban skies.

Was he a terrorist?? I don't know!! BUT,
before security could check,
he had left the place.
After I stood and loudly proclaimed,
"No one here, is carrying <u>your</u> case!"
(This was just after Lockabee.)

A romantic vacation package?
Why, that's every couple's dream.
We found some accommodations,
were not exactly what they seemed:

The *Cute Little Cottage*? Who could ask for more?
Uninvited Night Crawlers, covered the bathroom floor.

Beware of the *Room-With-A-View*?
It was next to the all-night Salsa bar!
If we only knew!
(My husband loves Mariachi Bands,
… or maybe **NOT!**)

No one spoke English in Mexico,
after *The Tourist Season.*
The Off-Season discount fairs,
were available for a reason.

Oh, who cares? We had fun, everywhere.
We were young and carefree.
Now, we laugh at it all;
yet, some leave *haunting* memories.

The little towns of dirt streets
with wooden planks for paths,
were like our old country towns
of our distant Western past.

Through the years, we've watched
many changes, to spare.
The dirt-road towns, "flowered" into
huge Tropical Town Squares.

The individual shops, where their goods
were made with care,
have given-way to co-op store fronts,
where the *Locals* sell their wares.

The small island airports, had
their dirt-floor shacks;
selling mementos of the Island's fame,
along with native snacks.

As tourism progressed, the tiny
dirt-floor airport rooms,
would turn into large Artistic Domes,
worthy of their booms.

Then, the cruise ships came;
with adventurous tourist, by the scores.
Now, the towns would need new buildings,
to house their Treasure Stores.

So, the tiny towns were looking ahead,
betting on their progress.
Do you think they ever wish to go back,
to those days of a slower past?

They are working so hard,
to give their tourist a peaceful rest.
I wonder if they might envy,
the solace of their guest.

What happens, when the "*Get-a-ways*" are gone?
How will we plan for that?
Shall we sing our *"Swans Song"* in another world,
or on a Distant Planet?

Like the many little dirt-road towns,
everything changes with time.
So, too, we go through metamorphosis, and,
I wouldn't change one moment of mine.

Sure, our fabric gets worn;
perhaps, tattered and threadbare.

Daily, we search for the parts that were torn,
and work on their repairs.

Everything has its' Ebbs and Flows;
we see it, with every glance.
Living each day to the fullest,
may yet, be your best defense.

There are so many textures;
I've listed, just a few.
Each one, a story unto itself.
(If you only knew!)

Adventures don't end with a disability.
I just find, what work's for me.
I may not remember all of my fun; but
a picture or friend will remind me of some.

Took the Glider Ride, for Mother's Day;
Soaring high currents, with the birds.
Dare to take a chance on life.
You need not miss its' worth.

I know *free glider rides* for Mothers,
may cause some families shame.
Would they think of it, as the movie,
"Throw Mama From The Train"?

It's more than the adventure;
all of the stories, are so unique.
This world-class pilot, told me all about,
her fascinating fetes…(Thanks Monique.)

Go ahead, tell me your life's stories.
I enjoy each and every one.
Many stories bring great laughter;
yet, a tear I shed for some.

I stand amazed by the bravery and valor;
that *Will* to overcome grief.
It gives you a whole new outlook,
on the quality of ones' beliefs.

The study of Nature and Human Nature,
brings solace to the soul.
Like Nature, living in peace and harmony,
might be a worthy goal.

Now, if all of these memories
are not good enough for me,
Then, just how ungrateful
would I be?

* * * * * * *

ADVENTURES

T0 BE CONTINUED

SIMPLY PUT:

IN A NUTSHELL, WHAT MY CONDITION IS LIKE.

%%%%%%%%%

MY TYPE OF SHORT-TERM MEMORY WAS
CAUSED BY A TRAUMATIC BRAIN INJURY.
(It works, or doesn't work, this way.) ☺

TODAY IS LOST IN A GOOD NIGHTS SLEEP.
SO, DON'T ASK ABOUT SOMETHING THAT
HAPPENED LAST WEEK!

REAMS OF PAPERS, I BRING WHEN WE MEET,
WILL GIVE YOU THE ANSWERS
TO THE QUESTIONS YOU SEEK!

I REALLY DON'T LIKE FEELING THIS MEEK,
SO, FOR FURTHER INSTRUCTIONS, PLEASE DOC!
WRITE IT DOWN ON A SHEET.

BETTER YET, DON'T EXPLAIN MY TEST RESULTS,
EXPECTING ME TO REMEMBER.
MY MEMORY IS A HINDER.

SEND HOME A COPY FOR MY PERSONAL USE.
FOR, KEEPING ME IN THE DARK,
THERE IS NO EXCUSE.

%%%%%%%%%

%%%%%%%%%

I HAVE A TYPE OF ATTENTION DEFICIT
WITH SLOWED ELOCUTION, WHICH WAS
CAUSED BY MY <u>NEAR-ELECTROCUTION</u>.
(It works, or doesn't work, this way:) ☺

MY HAND/EYE COORDINATION IS A LITTLE AMIS.
HOW DOES ONE EXPLAIN SOMETHING LIKE THIS?

ALL INCOMING STIMULI, WILL BE SLOWED;
THOSE TURN-AROUND REACTIONS WILL BE, ALSO.

I MUST CHANGE MY MODE, WITH EVERY NEW
SUBJECT.
IT'S ONLY A FEW SECONDS; SO YOU MAY NOT
DETECT IT.

HOWEVER, FAST MENTAL EXERCISES,
I WILL FIND QUITE TIRING.
ALL BECAUSE OF THIS BRAINS'
BURNED WIRING.

%%%%%%%%%

MEANWHILE, <u>INSIDE</u> THE NUTSHELL:

Fortunately, acceptance and learning to work with these disabilities, have made my Abilities strong enough to cover my Disabilities, usually. So, I'm okay with me.

ONE FACT REMAINS:

Our entire life is filled with choices. We start in our childhood, learning to make the right choices; what works for us, and what doesn't; what is socially acceptable, what is not; following the rules and laws, or facing the consequences, etc.

As we grow in years, the wisdom gleaned from our youth, settles into reality with the ability to check the variables and the logical outcome. Somewhere along the way, we have learned that: When we come to that Fork In The Road, we must choose left or right. Sometimes, the difference between the two, is just the matter of one little vowel: Our choices can leave us BITTER or make our life BETTER! I will always choose the latter; how about you? **HAVE A NICE LIFE !**

* * * * * * *

SURE, WE'VE RETIRED! Just for fun, I'm leaving a poem for others. The older we get, the faster time flies. (Or, do we slow down?) At any rate, we can't find enough time to do all of the things we want to do. Let's investigate why!

(Though, I would have shared their ambivalence about retirement. The not give up those surprise visits, or chances to see family and friends, anytime! Just, let us know when.)

* * * * * * *

NOW, I'M RETIRED !!!!

Yippee! I've never felt so free.
I don't have to be anyplace, I don't want to be.
I can even wear walk shorts, with my nubby knees.
'Cause, all the other gaffers, look a lot like me.

We bought a little home, just right for us.
We'll design our own garden, like we discussed.
I've bought the lawnmower, feeder, spreader, shovel,
wheelbarrow, fertilizer, planting soil, and anti-weed.

You bought the flowering fruit trees, rose bushes,
plants, and ground cover; to save time for me.
(Are you sure, that's what we agreed?)

I still have the ladder I bought,
for changing light bulbs.
"What's wrong with the color
of this house; it's brand new?"

(If I fell, it would likely be
into one of those beds of bulbs.)
"You've got to be kidding!
A weather vane on the flue?"

At times, my Tennis Elbows, Skiers Knees,
And Football Shoulders, bother me.
But, since there are no pressing tasks,
I can always take a little rest.

The yard sale went well, I must admit.
I'll let someone else do this work,
with the money I get.
The landscaping looks good,
someone will cut my grass,
while I just sit back and sip from my glass.

The weather vane did work quite well.
She was not wrong.
I'm not sure which direction the wind came from,
But we did have wind, 'cause the vane?
Well, It's gone!
Maybe the vane was in vain, like I said, but
I won't say a thing, if I treasure my head.

Doing all of this work, is like my old *"Nine to Five."*
If I keep up this pace, I will never survive.
I may take up golf, or play cards with the guys.
The girls are off shopping, looking at *"Great Buys!"*

It's just as we like it, our cozy little home.
With all of our leisure time, we are now free to roam.
Bought mountain bikes, to see what's around.
Hiked Nature Parks, where beauty abounds.

I must say, "We are having a ball!
Enjoying the pictures of things that we see;
we gave up traffic and Malls.
Now, we seek nature, flowers and trees.

Retiring is wonderful.
We've learned to relax and enjoy.
We visit the art museums, when traffic is light.
No crowds at the beaches, when weekdays are
bright.

There are weekend getaways, just for we two.
A leisurely time to choose, what we want to do.
A Theme Park or Water Park may be to our liking.
Then again, we can always go back to biking.

Grab a canoe trip, drifting down some scenic place.
How about a boat trip, with just a "One-Tank Dive?
Count the variety of Marine Life at our Inner Space.
Easy-going Scuba makes one feel so alive.

It's been a full weekend, there is no doubt.
Homeward bound! I'm tired and happy,
but just worn-out.

We'll drop off our luggage and
start a load of clothes.
Then we'll hit some Early Bird;
followed by a restful doze.
(We can really use that!)

But Wait! Is that the kids' van we see in our drive?!
If it's our kids, then they have kids….

"Grandma! Grandma! We came to surprise you."
(Oh, I'm surprised!!!)

"What are you fixing for supper? We're starved."
"We know a great place, where
your Dad can take us all to eat.
It isn't far, so go wash-up;
'cause we are also starved.
Grandma will cook tomorrow,
when she is not so *beat*."

"Grandma, why are you and Granddad *"draggin?"*
Dad says you're retired, and he's been bragging.
He knew you would like a great big surprise.
You have nothing to do, without us guys."

"Which room do you want us to go to sleep in?
We'll need an early start for Disney in the morning.
We're all going to Disney World,
(Without any warning?)
Then, we'll try a Water Park Slide,
just for some extra fun."

(How about sleeping in your room at home?)
(An early start? I'll do good to get my heart to start!)
(Disney World? You try the rides, we'll watch the movies.)
(I know his heart won't take that cold water slide.
In these hot temperatures,
it would be worse than the rides.)

"Disney World was so much fun,
we should all go back again!
Everyone did surprisingly well;
things moved very fast.

The lightening seen from the ferris wheel,
was really such a *blast!*
The downpour helped us all cool down.
Granddad was just as funny as a clown,
when he grabbed at his chest and
gulped that little pill down."

"This was one *cool* day; great fun!
I think we can all agree.
We'll bathe and take a quick nap.
We don't want to be in her way.
Because this is the day Grandma
wanted to cook for me,
And I can hardly wait. You know,
My Grandma's cooking is so great!"

Just two more days: Our son promises us
dinner-out everyday.
Breakfast and Lunch is nothing,
while the kids are at play.
Our pool is getting a work-out,
between the meals and hiking.
The parents are taking the kids out,
and we're resting to our liking.

"Mom and Dad have to go back to work
and we're still in school.
Maybe, when school is out…." Christmas for sure!
Right now, Granddad and I will be in school,
taking a Spanish Class.
"Mom! When did you sign-up for that?
You forgot to tell me this."

Well as we get older, they claim that we should
learn a foreign language, to preserve our mind.
The way things are going lately;
I think we're just-in-time.

ALWAYS LEAVE THEM LAUGHING!

WINDY WYNN

A SPECIAL THANKS TO ALL OF THE PEOPLE

WHO CARED ENOUGH TO MAKE A DIFFERENCE:

YOUR PRAYERS AND ENCOURAGEMENT WERE APPRECIATED.

Especially, TO MY HUSBAND VICTOR FOR ALL OF HIS CONSTANT HELP, PATIENCE, UNDERSTANDING, AND ENCOURAGEMENT. And TO MY SONS, MARK & WESLEY WYNN FOR "BEING THERE."

AND, For all of the peanut vendors everywhere.

THANKS, AGAIN !!

WINDY WYNN